"THE PHARMER'S ALMANAC"

A Training Manual on the Pharmacology
of Psychoactive Drugs

By:
Anthony B. Radcliffe, M.D.
Carol Forror Sites, Pharm.D
Peter A. Rush, Pharm.D
Joe Cruse, M.D.

Published by
M.A.C.
Printing and Publications Division
1850 High Street
Denver, Colorado 80218

CONTENTS

INTRODUCTION

The Pharmer's Almanac is designed to help teach non-medically trained professionals about the drugs on which people become dependent or addicted. Although statistics are difficult to interpret, the use of these drugs is involved in more deaths between the ages of 15 and 40 years than any other single cause. Science is not often mixed with the clinical decisions of day to day counseling and many counselors and nurses consider pharmacology the province of a very few. Our hope is to make this subject understandable and useable for counselors in helping treat chemically dependent patients.

Drug dependency is a psychic state and sometimes also a physical state resulting from the interaction between a living organism and a chemical (psychoactive drug) characterized by behavioral and other responses that always include a compulsion to take the chemical on a continuous or periodic basis in order to experience its psychic effects and sometimes to avoid the discomfort of its absence. In this book drug addiction is considered the severest presentation of drug dependency and is defined as a state of periodic or chronic intoxication, detrimental to the individual and society, produced by repeated consumption of the drug. It is usually characterized by a compulsion to take the drug (or a strong craving), by a tendency to increase the amount consumed, and by a set of signs and symptoms known as withdrawal, upon cessation of the drug.

We encourage those of you who may read this almanac to write and let us know if you find it helpful.

Learn and enjoy.

CHAPTER 1

Background

CHAPTER ONE

BACKGROUND

Throughout this book, key terms will be underlined and described when introduced. These underlined words are also defined in the appendix.

A. PHARMACOLOGY AND BIOPHARMACEUTICS

There are two areas of study which describe the actions of a drug. The first is how the drug affects the body. This area is called pharmacology.

Pharmacology studies the effects of a drug on the body in general as well as the drug effect on each organ, organ system, and individual cell.

The second area studies how the body processes drugs. This field is called biopharmaceutics, and is subdivided into four different categories: absorption, distribution, metabolism, and excretion.

Absorption deals with how the drug gets into the main blood circulation. When a drug is taken orally, it must be absorbed from the gastroin-

ABSORPTION: Entering Circulation

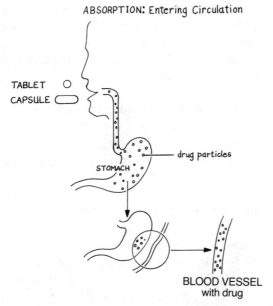

TABLET
CAPSULE

drug particles

STOMACH

BLOOD VESSEL
with drug

testinal tract (food processing system). When a drug is injected into a muscle or subcutaneously (just under the skin) it must be absorbed from these tissues into the main circulation. The major hindrances to absorption are the <u>membranes</u> that line the gastrointestinal tract, or the membranes in the tissue. Membranes are made up of lipid (fatty) substances. If a drug is not lipid soluble, it will not be able to cross through membranes. Thus it will not gain access to the blood-stream and will not reach the target organs. If a drug is injected intravenously, it does not need to be absorbed since it enters the blood circulation immediately. Most drugs of abuse are lipid soluble and can pass through the membranes necessary for absorption into the blood system.

The second phase of biopharmaceutics involves distribution of the drug within the body. Drugs usually do not distribute evenly throughout the whole body. The body tissues or organs have varying degrees of attraction for different drugs so that certain organs may have very high drug concentrations while other organs are almost devoid of drug. One area in the body which is difficult for a drug to gain entrance to is the brain. Also, simply entering the circulation does not guarantee that a drug will be active. It must also be in free form with access to the cells of the body. Many times, when a drug enters the blood, large quantities of it bind to proteins or fats in the blood or other parts of the body. While the drug exists in this bound form, it is unavailable to affect the body organs and cells. In time drugs of this type gradually unbind, and then are able to exert their action. Distribution is an important area to study since, if the range of distribution is known, the range of organs affected by the drug can also be determined.

The third area is metabolism and this may be the most important of the four subdivisions since this is an important mechanism that the body uses to alter drug action. Drug metabolism is the various chemical reactions involved in the transformation of a drug in the body usually from an active to an inactive compound. Sometimes drugs are metabolized to active compounds. Drug molecules can have parts removed or parts added to them in an attempt to alter the drug action or to create a molecule which is more water soluble so it will not cross membranes in the body. Water soluble drugs, or metabolites are more easily excreted via the urine. Metabolism in the body is accomplished with the aid of <u>enzymes</u> which are protein molecules that act as <u>catalysts</u> in biochemical reactions. Enzymes are found throughout the body, but the greatest concentration of enzymes are found in the liver. The liver then, is the area where the majority of drug metabolism occurs. When a drug is changed by the liver in this manner, the resultant products are called "metabolites". Metabolites may have the same or slightly reduced ability as the parent drug to cause an action. The metabolites may also sometimes be capable of producing a new (and sometimes undesirable) drug action. Usually, however, drug metabolites are incapable of causing a drug action and they are merely being made ready for excretion.

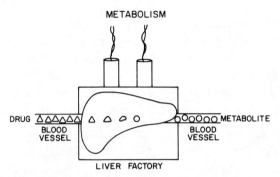

Excretion is the fourth and final phase of biopharmaceutics, and as the name implies, it deals with the elimination of the drug and its metabolites from the body. There are many routes of excretion from the body: expired air, tears, sweat, bile, urine, and feces. Probably the most common route of excretion is through urine.

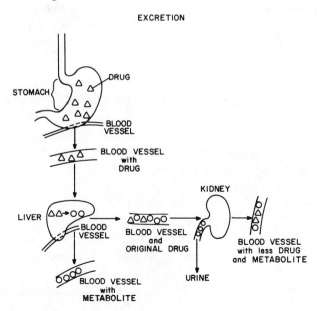

For a drug to be excreted in the urine, it needs to be water soluble (capable of being dissolved in water). A degree of water solubility can be inherent in the drug to begin with, or during metabolism, the drug can be made more water soluble. If a drug is somewhat water soluble to begin with, little or no metabolism is needed before excretion can occur.

SUMMARY

—Pharmacology — deals with the drug effects on the body.
—Biopharmaceutics — deals with the body's processing of drugs.
  —Absorption — is the process which gets a drug into the main circulation.
  —Distribution — describes parts of the body in which a drug concentrates.
  —Metabolism — basically, is the inactivation of a drug.
  —Excretion — method of ridding the drug from the body.

Drugs are chemicals which when swallowed, snorted, injected, or absorbed, through the skin, enter into a complex system. What ever their entry, they need to be broken down to active molecules, sent throughout the system where they will exert an action and eventually be rendered inactive and eliminated from the body. Alcohol, for example, is swallowed, gets into the bloodstream, goes to the brain where it helps to relax a person and then is degraded in the liver and eliminated. Psychoactive drugs are those drugs which exert an effect on the brain, many of which can become dependent or addicted to. These drugs easily get into a person's brain because they dissolve in fat tissue which is the primary substance of which our brain is composed.

B. BIOLOGICAL HALF-LIFE OF DRUGS (T1/2)

The biological half-life of a drug, abbreviated as T1/2, is the amount of time it takes for the body to eliminate half of the drug molecules from the blood stream. For instance, methadone has a T1/2 of about 24 hours. This means that 24 hours after taking a dose of methadone, the body will have eliminated 50% of the methadone molecules from the blood, thus leaving 50%. In the next 24 hours, half of the remaining methadone molecules will be eliminated, leaving 25% of the original dose. This process continues until the drug (from a single dose) is essentially completely eliminated.

HALF-LIFE

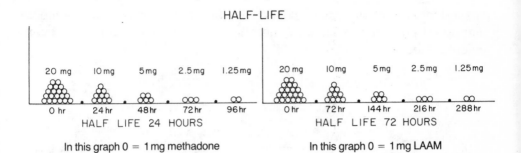

HALF LIFE 24 HOURS

In this graph 0 = 1 mg methadone

HALF LIFE 72 HOURS

In this graph 0 = 1 mg LAAM

Understanding the half-life of a drug can allow one to better know how long the drug may have an effect. Keep in mind that a patient may not feel the effects of a drug any longer, even before the first T1/2 is reached. This does not mean that there is no drug left, but that there is insufficient drug to cause an effect. However, there may be enough drug left to interact with other drugs, producing an unexpected effect, if the second drug is taken while the first is still present in sufficient quantity.

C. LIVER

The liver is one of the main "processing plants" in the body. It is involved with the storage, building, and breakdown of carbohydrates (groups of substances such as sugars and starches containing carbon, hydrogen, and oxygen), fats and proteins. When the body builds or breaks down chemicals in this way, it is called metabolism or biotransformation.

When a drug enters the body, it also will be metabolized, or changed by the liver. Four things may happen when the liver changes a drug:
1. An active drug is changed to a compound which no longer causes any effect in the body (most common occurrence).
2. An active drug is degraded into other active metabolites.
3. An inactive compound which has no effect on the body is changed into an active metabolite.
4. An inactive compound is changed to another inactive compound and is excreted. (Obviously not a desirable drug!)

The liver, then is basically an organ where a potentially dangerous compound is made into a less dangerous one. In the liver the main metabolizing areas are inside the cells in places called <u>microsomes</u>. Within the microsomes are proteins called enzymes. Enzymes are compounds which aid in the chemical reactions which form the breakdown products, (called metabolites). Enzymes exist all over the body, however, the most important enzymes for general metabolism are those found in the liver microsomes.

METABOLISM IN LIVER CELL MICROSOME

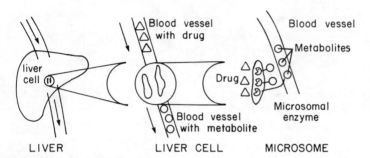

In this illustration, from left to right, a liver cell is enlarged, revealing microsomes, then a microsome is enlarged, revealing enzymes exerting their action on the drug.

LIVER   LIVER CELL   MICROSOME

The microsomal enzymes, and therefore metabolism itself, can be affected by age, condition of the liver, concommittant disease, and by exposure to drugs. The very young and very old do not have as many microsomal enzymes as healthy adults between the ages of about 15 and 60 years. People with liver disease, such as cirrhosis also do not have as many microsomal enzymes. In these people the metabolism of drugs may be slowed and continuous dosing can lead to greater drug effect, due to less metabolism to inactive products. Also if an inactive drug which needs to be metabolized to become active is given, we would expect it to have less of an effect.

Certain drugs can also affect the enzyme systems in the liver. The most common occurrence is where repeated usage of the drug stimulates the production of more of the enzymes used in its own breakdown. This means there are more enzymes available to degrade the drug so that the drug is metabolized faster than usual; therefore the drug effect will be shorter than expected. This process is called enzyme induction and occurs with certain drugs, especially sedative hypnotic drugs; such as alcohol, barbiturates, etc. If another drug uses these same enzymes, its length of action will also be reduced, creating a drug interaction. This is the basis for tolerance, where it would take more of a drug to produce the same effect.

After absorption of a drug from the stomach or intestines, the blood carrying the drug must pass through the liver first before going to the rest of the body. Much of the drug can be degraded by this passage through the liver (called the "first pass effect"). If these drugs can reach the main circulation without going through the liver — for instance, if they enter the blood by being absorbed through the skin, or by being injected just beneath the skin layer or into the muscle, or by being absorbed through nasal membranes or the lung, the effect of the drug will be seen sooner.

The breakdown products formed by the liver from any particular drug can go through many different changes. The process of metabolizing is not always detoxifying, since a metabolite can be formed which is more toxic than the parent compound, and this can be quite dangerous. Usually the end result of metabolism though, is to make a compound which is more water soluable than the parent compound, and therefore easier to pass in the urine. This is most frequently done by adding of small water-like groups or large water soluble groups to the drug molecule.

D. KIDNEY

The kidney is one of the main disposal sites for liquid substances in the body. Blood passes through the kidney and it filters the blood and removes water soluble waste particles. When a drug is in the body, it will be filtered out of the blood when it reaches the kidney. Once inside the kidney, the drug will travel down little hollow tubules where the contents are processed for removal. These tubules are lined with fat cells (have lipid walls) and are surrounded by blood vessels. If the drugs or other compounds in the tubules are fat (lipid) soluble, they can pass through the fat walls and re-enter the main blood circulation and the drug effect may re-occur.

This is why the liver is so important in the excretion of many drugs. The liver's main drug metabolizing function is to create a compound which is water soluble. The more water soluble a metabolite is (and therefore the less lipid soluble it is) the harder it will be for it to pass through the lipid tubule wall in the kidney and get back into the blood stream. A highly water soluble molecule must then remain in the tubule and eventually become part of the urine which is excreted.

SUMMARY:

—Biological half-life- is the amount of time it takes for the body to eliminate half of the drug molecules from the blood stream.
—The liver- can be depicted as a processing factory.

—Microsomes- are major areas in the liver cells where drug metabolism occurs.

—Enzymes- involved in drug metabolism are found in high concentration in the microsomes.

—Enzyme induction and tolerance- occur when repeated usage of a drug causes an increase in enzyme activity.

—"First pass" effect- is metabolism which occurs when medications taken by mouth pass through the liver before going to the rest of the body.

—The kidney- acts as a disposal system for water soluble substances.

If 10mg of Valium® is taken on Monday at 9:00AM, only 5mg will be eliminated by Tuesday at 9:00AM. This means there is 5mg of Valium® available to be active. This may produce no effect but if alcohol were ingested during this period the combination of the alcohol plus the Valium® could cause the person to go to sleep permanently. This unexpected effect is called synergism and usually occurs in people who have been taking sleeping pills, alcohol, or tranquilizers over a long time.

E. BLOOD BRAIN BARRIER

The brain is surrounded by several membranes as well as the blood vessel walls of the arteries which supply the brain with blood. These membranes and vessel walls set up a barrier around the brain that is selective as to what can cross over into the brain tissue from the main blood circulation. This is called the blood brain barrier (BBB).

The types of molecules which have the best chance of crossing over into the brain tissue are those that are lipid (fat) soluble, since the barrier is composed mainly of lipid compounds. Psychoactive drugs can cross over very easily and their brain tissue concentrations increase significantly. Other drugs cannot cross this blood brain barrier at all, and therefore no central nervous system effect will be seen. Most drugs which people become dependent on or addicted to are lipid soluble to some extent and can cross into the brain. As the liver metabolizes these drugs, however, they become more water soluble and less lipid soluble. This means that the metabolites will have less and less of a chance to cross the blood brain barrier and a greater chance to be excreted.

F. NERVES AND NEUROTRANSMITTERS

The central nervous system (CNS) is that part of the nervous system which includes the brain and the spinal cord. The rest of the nerves, including the nerves which go out from the brain to the peripheral areas, such as those which take care of touch, feeling, and muscle coordination are part of the peripheral nervous system.

The parts of the body are in constant communication with the brain. This is accomplished by networks of nerves some of which carry messages up to and back from the brain. A particular nerve is made up of several nerve cells stretched out in a line of communication from the brain to a particular part of the body. It used to be thought that the communication along the nerve was accomplished all by means of electrical activity. It is now known that this theory is only partly true. Electrical transmission does occur within each nerve cell, but some other means is needed to jump the "gap" between the individual nerve cells. The gap between nerve cells is called a synapse. Since electrical transmission cannot occur through the synapse, the cells continue their communication by little chemical messengers called neurotransmitters sent out into the space (synapse). A nerve cell will electrically generate a message along its length until it reaches a synapse. This end of the nerve is referred to as the pre-synaptic nerve ending. At the synapse little packets of chemicals called neurotransmitters are released which carry the message over the gulf to the next nerve cell called the post-synaptic nerve ending. The neurotransmitters then briefly bind to the post-synaptic nerve ending and stimulate an electrical impulse that is generated down that nerve to the next synapse.

Once the neurotransmitters have been released and have carried their message across the synapse, they may be taken back up into the nerve from which they were released and "repackaged" for release again or they may be destroyed by enzymes which are found in the synaptic gulf. The most important of these enzymes are monoamine oxidase (MAO), catechol-O-methyltransferase (COMT), and acetylcholine esterase (AChase). The message carried by neurotransmitters is stopped by one of these two methods so that new messages carried by other neurotransmitter molecules can then proceed.

There are many types of neurotransmitters in the body. Some of the most important with respect to psychoactive drugs are norepinephrine,

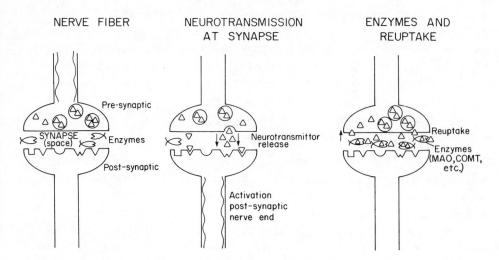

dopamine, acetylcholine, GABA (gamma-amino-butyric acid) and serotonin (also called 5-hydroxytryptamine or 5-HT).

The neurotransmitter system in the CNS is separate from the neurotransmitter systems in the rest of the body. In other words, just because
something works a particular way in the peripheral nervous system and
body, it does not necessarily mean it will work that way in the CNS, and
visa versa. It is very important to remember that the CNS operates under
a different set of "rules" than does the rest of the body and the CNS and
periphery should be considered as two separate systems.

SUMMARY:

—The blood brain barrier- prevents most drugs from entering the brain.
Psychoactive drugs can cross into the brain.
—The CNS- consists of nerves of the brain and spinal cord.
   —A synapse- is the small gap between nerve cells where many
chemicals exert their effects.
—Neurotransmitters- are the chemicals which transmit nerve messages
across the synapse.

Actually very few drugs get into the brain. This is because the brain is
protected by a barrier of tissue which keeps most drugs out such as
antibiotics or heart medicines. Drugs on which people become dependent or addicted can easily get into the brain because they can pass
through fat tissue. (This is what is meant by lipid solubility.)

Most functions in the brain are finely tuned by special chemicals called neurotransmitters. These substances interact with nerve cells to get us fired up or calmed down. Many of the psychoactive drugs stimulate the release of these neurotransmitters which then cause wakefulness or sleep.

G. CELL RECEPTOR THEORY

For a drug to have an effect, it must react with body components. The site of action of drugs is at the cellular level. Most drugs attach by means of chemical binding to specific sites located either on the outer membranes of the cell, or in its interior. These specific places where drugs bind to the cell are called receptor sites. Once the drug binds to the receptor site, it will cause a change in the normal workings of that cell. This, then, leads to the observed drug effect. The drug effect is proportionate to the number of drug molecules which bind to the cell receptors — that is, the more drug-to-cell binding which occurs, the greater the drug effect.

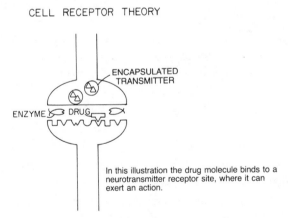

CELL RECEPTOR THEORY

In this illustration the drug molecule binds to a neurotransmitter receptor site, where it can exert an action.

Many different types of cells may be capable of binding the same drug, but the changes within the cells evoked by the binding may be completely different. For instance, a drug bound to one cell may cause blood vessel dilation (widening), whereas the same drug bound to a different type of cell may cause blood vessel constriction (narrowing). Also, a particular cell may have receptor sites for many different drugs — each of which could cause a different cellular change. The total drug effect, then, will be the sum of all the cells affected.

The binding of a drug to a cell receptor is reversible, therefore as metabolism and excretion remove the drug from circulation, there become fewer drug molecules left to bind with the receptors and the drug effect diminishes.

H. AUTONOMIC NERVOUS SYSTEM

The autonomic nervous system is the part of the nervous system which controls various automatic functions such as heart rate, digestive processes, etc. The autonomic nervous system is divided into two parts: the sympathetic nervous system (SNS) and the parasympathetic nervous system (PSNS). These two divisions work together to form a proper balance of function within the body.

The SNS is called the "fight or flight" system. It is the system which dominates during stressful situations. If you picture a body preparing it for some sort of action — e.g. a soldier going into battle, a runner readying for a race — it is easy to understand the changes which occur with SNS domination. First, the heart rate and respiratory rate will increase and airways will open wide to increase the availability of oxygen to brain, muscle, and other cells. Blood vessels in the skin and peripheral areas will constrict while blood vessels in the heart, brain, muscle and other vital areas will dilate so the blood will go where it is most needed. Digestive processes, including salivation, all but stop so that energy need not be wasted there. Pupils of the eyes will dilate to allow maximal vision, and the eyes will adjust to distant vision.

The PSNS, on the other hand, acts in an opposite manner to the SNS. The PSNS is sometimes called the "feed and breed" system. As this description implies, this system is involved with the normal daily functionings of the body. The PSNS causes a slowing of the heart and respiratory rates. Body secretions such as saliva and tears are stimulated, and digestive processes are carried out. Urination and defecation can occur, whereas during SNS dominance, the muscles controlling these processes are tightly constricted. The pupils of the eye constrict and the eyes are adjusted for close vision.

The SNS uses two neurotransmitters to carry its messages to the various organs. These neurotransmitters are called norepinephrine and epinephrine. Epinephrine is also called adrenalin so the SNS is sometimes also referred to as the adrenergic nervous system. The PSNS uses only one neurotransmitter to carry its messages and that neuro-transmitter is acetylcholine. The PSNS is, therefore, also called the cholinergic nervous system. The SNS and the PSNS usually work in balance to establish the best working condition for the body for any particular situation. This balance can be broken, however by manipulation with drugs, or by various disease states. SNS domination can be achieved by two different methods: either the direct stimulation of the SNS or by suppression of the PSNS. In like fashion, the PSNS can become dominant either by direct stimulation or by suppression of the SNS. Drugs which stimulate the SNS are called sympathomimetics (they "mimic" the SNS effects) and drugs which suppress the SNS are called sympatholytics ("lysis" means breaking down).

Drugs which affect the PSNS are called cholinergics (drugs which act in a manner similar to acetylcholine) or anticholinergics (drugs which antagonize the action of acetylcholine). Thus to achieve SNS dominance, the sympathomimetics (to stimulate the SNS) or anticholinergics (to suppress the PSNS) can be used. Also, to obtain PSNS dominance, cholinergics or sympatholytics can be used. The drugs of abuse which affect the autonomic nervous system are usually those which cause SNS dominance.

AUTONOMIC BALANCE

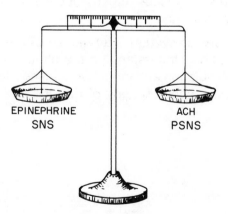

EPINEPHRINE   ACH
SNS   PSNS

Examples of some sympathomimetics which are frequently abused are the amphetamines and cocaine. Examples of some anticholinergic drugs are atropine (and other belladonna derived compounds such as those found in Contac® cold capsules and jimson weed). These drugs and principles will be discussed in detail later.

SYSTEM	TRANSMITTER/DRUG	EFFECT
SNS	Norepinephrine, Epinephrine	Stimulation-SNS Dominance
SNS	Amphetamine, Cocaine	Stimulation-SNS Dominance
PSNS	Acetylcholine	Stimulation-PSNS Dominance
PSNS	Atropine	Antagonism-SNS Dominance
PSNS	Glutethimide (Doriden®)	Antagonism-SNS Dominance
PSNS	Chlorpromazine (Thorazine®)	Antagonism-SNS Dominance

SUMMARY:

—The autonomic nervous system- controls many of the maintenance functions of the body.

—The sympathetic nervous system- is also known as the "fight or flight" system, and controls the body's response to stress. Its neurotransmitters are epinepherine, and norepinephrine. Drugs which affect it are either sympathomimetics or sympatholytics.

—The parasympathetic nervous system- is also known as the "feed or breed" system. In many ways it works opposite to the sympathetic nervous system. Its neurotransmitter is acetylcholine and drugs which affect it are either cholinergics or anticholinergics.

Most drugs have their effect in the body by binding to some part of a body cell. Drug action continues until the individual drug molecules are metabolized and/or excreted.

The autonomic nervous system is a key part of the body where many drugs exert their action. Understanding the effects of sympathetic and parasympathetic stimulation and inhibition are important to understanding the effects on the body of many of the drugs of abuse.

CHAPTER 2

Sedative-Hypnotic Drugs

SEDATIVE-HYPNOTIC-DRUGS

Sedative-hypnotic drugs (SHD's) represent all tranquilizers, sleeping pills, alcohol, anesthetics, and antihistamines. Alcohol, barbiturates, benzodiazepines, and other sedative-hypnotic drugs are considered a single pharmacological category of central nervous system depressants or "downers." They are characterized by the following:

1. Increasing dosages produce signs of progressive central nervous system depression ranging from sedation to sleep.
2. Overdose will cause mental clouding, loss of muscular coordination, and eventually respiratory arrest.
3. Chronic use of high doses leads to the development of tolerance, but a level of intoxication can always be reached if the dose is high enough.
4. There is cross tolerance between the groups: for instance, an alcoholic may be somewhat tolerant to the effects of sleeping pills or tranquilizers.
5. Chronic use of large doses leads to physical dependence and withdrawal if usage is abruptly stopped. Withdrawal symptoms can be lessened to a certain extent if a drug from another class of sedatives is substituted. For instance, an alcoholic may be able to stop withdrawal by substituting barbiturates during his alcohol withdrawal.
6. When drugs from this class are taken together one sees a far greater CNS depressant effect than otherwise would be expected. This is called synergism.

The drugs to be discussed in this section, then, will be: A. Alcohol; B. The Barbiturates; C. The Benzodiazepines (Valium®, Librium®, etc.); D. Miscellaneous Sedatives (such as Quaalude®, Chloral Hydrate®, meprobamate, and others).

CHAPTER TWO-A

ALCOHOL:

1. <u>EPIDEMIOLOGY</u> (The study of spreading of disease).

Alcohol, and other drug dependancies are the major health problems among young adults and adolescents. The costs in life, health, and property, attributable to alcohol alone are staggering.

The annual per capita consumption of alcohol (also known as <u>ethanol</u> or ethyl alcohol) in Americans above the age of 15 is 2.65 gallons. (This figure represents pure alcohol, and is equal to about 707 twelve ounce cans of beer per year.) This ranges from 3.1 gallons (827 cans of beer) per person on the Pacific coast, down to 1.81 gallons (483 cans of beer) per person in the heart of the South East. This compares with the French rate of 6.53 gallons per person per year (1,741 cans of beer), and the Israeli 0.82 gallons per person per year (219 cans of beer). Probably around 10 million Americans suffer from alcohol dependency or addiction. Cirrhosis of the liver, which usually results from chronic alcoholism, is the sixth most common cause of death in the U.S. In addition to the morbidity resulting from the disease process of alcohol dependency (which we will look at in more detail later) there are accidents and crimes resulting in injuries and fatalities.

—Of the 51,093 deaths in motor vehicles in 1979, 50% of the drivers had been drinking.

—Of the 2,609,000 injuries in motor vehicles in 1979, 30% of the drivers had been drinking.

—50% of all fatal falls involve people who had been drinking.

—68% of all drowning victims (and 85% of all adult drowning victims) had been drinking.

—Alcohol is involved in: 64% of homocides, 75% of stabbings, 55% of shootings, 69% of beatings, 30% of all suicides, 55% of all arrests, 67% of sexually agressive acts against children, 30% of sexually agressive acts against women, and 56% of all fights or assaults in the home.

2. BIOPHARMACEUTICS

ABSORPTION.

Alcohol is readily and passively absorbed along the entire length of the gastrointestinal system. Usually about 20% of the ingested alcohol will be absorbed from the stomach while the other 80% is absorbed from the first portion of the small intestine. If there is food in the stomach, it can delay the usual 20% absorption of alcohol from the stomach. Also, food in the stomach causes a delay to occur in the emptying of the stomach contents into the intestines since the food must be partially digested by the stomach first. This will cause a delay in the alcohol reaching the small intestines where the maximum alcohol absorption occurs. Thus, alcohol will be more slowly absorbed on a full stomach, and with less absorption, there will be less effect. If the stomach is empty, alcohol will be absorbed quite rapidly and blood levels will rise suddenly. This is why it is so much easier to feel the effects of alcohol on an empty stomach.

Carbonated drinks (such as champagne) are also absorbed quite fast, since they probably stimulate the stomach to empty its contents into the small intestine where alcohol is more completely and rapidly absorbed.

DISTRIBUTION.

Alcohol is a very simple molecule because it only contains two carbon atoms: CH_3-CH_2-OH. It is a small water soluble molecule and once it is absorbed, it goes everywhere that blood goes, so that it has the potential of affecting every organ in the body. Alcohol readily passes through the blood brain barrier, as well, since it is lipid soluble and such a small molecule. Alcohol can affect children of alcoholic mothers, because it easily crosses the placental barrier and fetal alcohol syndrome (FAS) can result. Some of the more prominent effects noted in FAS are: low birth weight and length, small head circumference, abnormal bone and tissue structures of the midfacial area, and mild to moderate mental retardation. Alcohol enters breast milk from the blood. When blood levels are high, or when alcohol is taken in high quantities for prolonged periods while a mother is breast feeding, intoxication can occur in the newborn. Also, when alcohol blood levels are high, the ability of mother's milk to flow is inhibited.

METABOLISM AND EXCRETION.

Most alcohol is metabolized and only a small amount (2-10%, depending on the quantity ingested) is eliminated unchanged in breath, urine, sweat, bile, or tears.

The main metabolite or breakdown product of alcohol is acetaldehyde and 85-90% of the metabolism occurs in the liver. Acetaldehyde is rapidly degraded to acetic acid which will eventually be broken down to carbon dioxide (CO_2) and water (H_2O). There are three basic enzyme systems involved in the metabolism of alcohol to acetaldehyde:

1. Alcohol dehydrogenase;
2. Microsomal ethanol oxidizing system (MEDS); and
3. Catalase system.

1. The alcohol dehydrogenase (ADH) pathway converts alcohol to acetaldehyde using the ADH enzyme plus an energy cofactor in the body called NAD (nicotinamide-adenine dinucleotide):

$$CH_3\text{-}CH_2\text{-}OH + NAD \xrightarrow{\text{Alcohol Dehydrogenase}} CH_3\text{-}CHO + NADH + H^+$$

Another enzyme, called acetaldehyde dehydrogenase, will then use another NAD energy molecule to change acetaldehyde to acetate.

$$CH_3\text{-}CHO + NAD + H_2O \xrightarrow{\text{Acetaldehyde Dehydrogenase}} CH_3\ COOH + NADH + H^+$$

ADH PATHWAY OF ALCOHOL METABOLISM

Acetaldehyde is a toxic compound. When present in sufficient quantity in the blood, it can cause: flushing, throbbing headache, nausea, vomiting, decreased blood pressure, thirst, and other reactions. A drug called disulfram (Antabuse®), blocks the conversion of acetaldehyde to acetate, resulting in higher levels of acetaldehyde in the blood. The reaction of acute toxic symptoms which is seen when alcohol is taken along with Antabuse®, is called the "Disulfram Ethanol Reaction" DER. This drug reaction is taken advantage of in therapy. Patients desiring to abstain from alcohol are often given Antabuse® to help them maintain abstinance.

$$CH_3\text{-}CHO + NAD + H_2O \longrightarrow CH_3\,COOH + NADH + H^{\oplus}$$

Acetaldehyde ⟵————— ANTABUSE®
Dehydrogenase

With both alcohol dehydrogenase and acetaldehyde dehydrogenase using up large quantities of NAD in their reactions, it is easy to see that with excessive alcohol intake, a lot of NAD molecules will be converted to NADH and the normal NAD/NADH ratio will be shifted from 5/5 to 1/9. Since the NAD energy molecule is involved in many other of the body's metabolic workings, the decrease of NAD and the increase of NADH could cause many problems in the body.

2. A second metabolic process for dealing with alcohol is the microsomal ethanol oxidizing system (MEOS). This process also requires an energy molecule in its reaction, called NADPH, which is converted during the reaction to NADP. The MEOS becomes more important in metabolizing alcohol after chronic alcohol use. Alcohol is again metabolized to acetaldehyde by these enzymes:

$$NADPH + CH_3\text{-}CH_2\text{-}OH + H^+ + O_2 \xrightarrow{MEOS} CH_3\text{-}CHO + NADP + H_2O$$

3. The third metabolic process for dealing with alcohol is called the catalase system. The catalase system also involves the use of NADPH plus the use of hydrogen peroxide. The participation of this pathway in the metabolism of alcohol is still questionable and may not be very important.

ADH is the primary system involved in alcohol metabolism. With infrequent drinking, the MEOS system accounts for perhaps 20-25% of the metabolism of alcohol, while the ADH system metabolizes the rest. However, with chronic alcohol use, the MEOS system may take on more importance, since these enzymes are stimulated to increase in number. This enzyme replication, also called enzyme induction may partially account for the development of tolerance to alcohol since there will be more enzymes to degrade the alcohol and therefore a shorter duration of action. Enzyme induction in response to alcohol is apparently under genetic control. As a result, enzyme induction is quite variable from person to person.

MEOS AND ENZYME INDUCTION

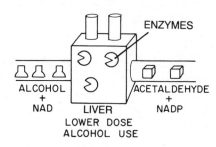

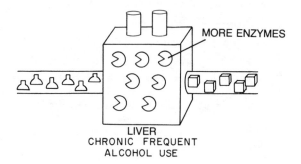

SUMMARY (Biopharmaceutics of Alcohol):

—The absorption of alcohol- is affected by the time it takes the stomach to empty its contents.
—Alcohol is distributed- to all parts of the body and is readily able to cross all membrane barriers.
—The metabolism of alcohol- occurs mainly in the liver.
   —ADH and MEOS- are the most important systems involved in the breakdown of alcohol to acetaldehyde.
   —DER- results from a build up of acetaldehyde, caused by a chemically induced block in its metabolism.

The reason for understanding the metabolism or breakdown of alcohol is because pharmacologists have developed drugs which interfere with this breakdown. (Antabuse® is the best known example.) When a person drinks, their body accumulates acetaldehyde, which causes nausea, vomiting, a decrease in blood pressure, facial flushing and an increase in body temperature.

3. PHARMACOLOGY

Many of the effects of ethanol, including those seen within peripheral systems such as the stomach, intestines, heart, and blood vessels are caused by actions somewhere in the brain.

One of the first parts of the brain that alcohol affects is the <u>reticular activating system</u> (RAS). The RAS is a portion of the brain stem which takes incoming peripheral nervous messages and deciphers them and weeds certain things out before sending the messages on up to the cortex. It then takes the messages coming back from the cortex and combines them and sends them to their appropriate areas. The RAS acts somewhat like a secretary screening and organizing the messages going to and coming from the boss.

The RAS can be divided into two parts — the stimulating component and the depressing component. When the stimulating component is dominant the message flow is good and a person is awake and function-

BALANCE OF NEUROTRANSMITTERS IN THE RAS

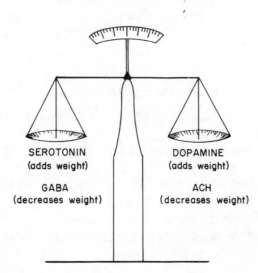

SEROTONIN
(adds weight)

DOPAMINE
(adds weight)

GABA
(decreases weight)

ACH
(decreases weight)

ing. If the depressive component is dominant, the message flow into, and therefore out of, the cortex is slowed and if it becomes slowed enough, the person will fall asleep. The body has a complex method for controlling this, involving four brain chemicals called neurotransmitters. These neurotransmitters are: dopamine, acetylcholine, serotonin, and GABA (gamma-amino butyric acid).

Alcohol causes the depressant side of the RAS to dominate by stimulating the release of dopamine. With sufficient alcohol intake muscular and neurologic reactions begin to malfunction, and thought becomes jumbled and disorganized, since the cortex is no longer receiving coordinated information from the RAS and since its messages are no longer flowing out accurately to the rest of the body.

The first mental processes to be affected are those that depend on training and previous experiences — the processes that usually make a person sober and exhibit self-restraint. Memory, concentration, and insight are first dulled then lost altogether. Confidence abounds, the person becomes vivacious and more talkative. Mood swings, however, are uncontrolled and emotional outbursts are frequent. As intoxication increases, there is a general decrease of nervous function until a person loses conciousness. The following table describes the relative physical and mental effects with a corresponding blood alcohol level.

Blood Alcohol Level-gm/100ml	Symptoms
.02-.09	Muscular incoordination, impaired sensory function and changes in mood, behavior and personality.
.10-.19	Mental impairment, incoordination and staggering.
.20-.29	Nausea, vomiting, double vision and marked staggering.
.30-.39	Decreased body temperature, severe speech problems and amnesia.
.40-.70	Coma, respiratory failure and death.

These blood levels and correlating physiological symptoms represent the effects seen in a non-tolerant individual. Blood alcohol level does not correlate well with the number of drinks inbibed. This is because other factors, including race, age, weight and sex of the individual, amount of alcohol contained in the drink, and length-of use may also affect the blood level. Also keep in mind that the effects based on blood alcohol level will vary with tolerance, sex of the individual, and other factors. A blood alcohol of 0.1 gm/100ml and above is considered the legal level for intoxication in most States in the USA.

In general, the effects of alcohol on the central nervous system (CNS) correspond with the levels of alcohol in the blood, however, the effects are more marked as the blood alcohol level is rising than when it is falling. In other words, a person may begin to have slurred speech at a blood level of 0.08gm/100ml as he is drinking, but after he quits drinking, he may return to normal speech while his blood level is still 0.1, but falling. This is called "acute tolerance" or tachyphylaxis since it occurs while a person is drinking and can occur even on initial exposure. It may or may not be related to chronic tolerance that occurs with longer term drinking.

With long term alcohol intake, a person does become tolerant to its effects so that progresssively higher amounts are used to achieve the same state of intoxication. Part of this tolerance may be due to the faster metabolism of the alcohol that is caused by induction of liver enzyme systems. This does not completely explain tolerance, however, since a chronic drinker could appear sober at a blood level that would make a naive drinker quite drunk. Therefore, there must be some mechanism within the brain itself which eventually adjusts to the chronic exposure of the brain to alcohol. It is also important to remember that the blood levels of alcohol and the corresponding degree of intoxication as shown in the table above which is gm/100ml correlated with symptoms will not be the same as with a tolerant person, except for the lethal limit. The lethal limit can increase slightly with tolerance, but it will not increase indefinitely.

Alcohol also affects normal sleeping patterns. Normal sleep consists of several different phases, one of which is called rapid eye movement (REM) sleep. REM sleep occurs during a period when there is rapid movement of the eyes under the closed lids. The REM sleep is usually associated with dreaming and its exact purpose is not clearly understood. It is known, however, that alcohol causes a decrease in the amount of time that is usually spent in REM sleep. However upon withdrawal from alcohol, the percentage of sleep devoted to REM sleep is increased dramatically. This is called "REM rebound" and the person experiences many unpleasant dreams and nightmares.

Up to now, what has been said about the basic mechanism of alcohol and the effects of increasing doses are basically true for all sedative hypnotics. However, certain effects occur in various tissues and organs of the body that are unique to alcohol alone. This occurs due to three mechanisms:

1. Alcohol can serve as a source of calories but does not provide a balanced diet. Vitamin and mineral deficiencies can occur due to this imbalance. Even with adequate diets, alcohol dependent persons have a decreased ability to absorb and utilize three important vitamins: B1 (thiamine), B12 (cyanocobalamine), and folic acid.

2. Alcohol and its metabolite acetaldehyde can have direct toxic effects on cells.

3. Alcohol affects normal metabolic functioning of the body by increasing the NAD/NADH ratio during the metabolism of alcohol by the ADH system.

PERIPHERAL NERVE DAMAGE

Damage of the nerves in the periphery causes numbness, especially in the legs. It varies from patchy loss of sensation in the feet to the loss of sensory perception in the entire leg. With this loss of sensation, an alcohol dependent person could hurt himself and not even be aware of it. Some people believe that this nerve damage is due to the loss of Vitamin B1; however B1 replacement therapy may not reverse the damage once it is done.

CNS CHANGES

1. Wernicke-Korsakoff Syndrome is a continuum of pathological changes which occur in the brain after chronic exposure to alcohol. Wernicke's syndrome is the earlier form. It is characterized by disorientation, peripheral nerve damage, loss of muscular coordination and involuntary, rapid horizontal eye movements (nystagmus) which can eventually progress to paralysis of all eye movements. A person with this problem will have to turn their head to see things which are to the side of their vision, since they cannot move their eyes.

Wernicke's syndrome is thought to be caused by a Vitamin B1 (thiamine) deficiency. If replacement therapy is not started, the mental state of the person may deteriorate with the appearance of marked confusion. Eventually Korsakoff's psychosis will appear. The person will experience periods of amnesia and will readily answer questions and relate experiences without regard to the accuracy of the matter. The memory impairment is so severe that a person will make up any kind of story — which they actually consider to be the truth — just to fill in the gaps. And the stories may change from minute to minute without the person noticing any inconsistencies. This is called confabulation. Korsakoff's psychosis is not as responsive to Vitamin B1 therapy as is the earlier Wernicke form and once this point has been reached, the damage is irreversible. Wernicke-Korsakoff Syndrome can occur in severe malnutrition without alcohol abuse, but it occurs in the U.S. almost exclusively in alcoholics.

2. Alcoholic dementia occurs while a person is going through alcohol withdrawal. It is characterized by disturbances of memory and thought content, confabulation, and loss of decorum. These symptoms may decrease with time and eventually disappear completely. However, some evidence of brain disorder will still remain, due to an actual loss of cells from the cortex, or the "thinking" portion of the brain. Autopsies of even relatively young alcoholics often show an unexpected wasting away of the brain, especially in the cortex region. At this time, this cortical wasting does not correlate with clinically observed effects.

GASTROINTESTINAL PROBLEMS

1. Stomach and small intestine:
High beverage alcohol concentration, from 20-80% (40-160 proof), causes an erosion of the stomach lining and also interferes with the body's attempt to repair the damage.

BEVERAGE-Amount	% Alcohol by volume	Proof (double %)	Gm alcohol/amount
Beer 12oz can	3-6	6-12	11-21
Table wine 4oz glass	12	24	14
Distilled spirits 1 oz shot: Whiskey, Rum, Gin, Vodka	35-80	70-160	10-24

Also, alcohol decreases the production of mucus in the gastrointestinal tract. This mucus serves as a protective lining and helps the stomach and intestinal lining from being broken down by digestive enzymes.

One of the most common signs of gastrointestinal disease associated with acute or chronic alcohol abuse is blood loss. The loss may be massive or not even visible to the naked eye, but it is usually due to the irritation to the stomach caused by the alcohol.

High alcoholic concentration also impairs the absorption of certain substances from the small bowel into the body. One of the compounds affected in this manner is Vitamin B1 and this is why chronic alcohol users run such high risk of being deficient in this vitamin.

2. Large Intestine:

Alcohol can affect the colon in two completely different manners. Constipation can occur with continuous alcohol use which is probably due to an inadequate bulk intake. On the other hand, diarrhea may occur, usually due to the irritating effect of the flavoring oils in the alcoholic beverage. In the chronic alcohol dependent person, diarrhea may also indicate vitamin deficiencies or chronic blood loss through the gastrointestinal tract.

LIVER

1. Fatty Liver:

It was explained before that the alcohol dehydrogenase (ADH) enzyme system increases the ratio of NADH to NAD. This increase in NADH causes an increase in the production of fatty compounds which are deposited in the liver. Alcohol-production of fats can also displace the use of normal dietary fats in the body so there is an even greater excess of fat in the liver if high alcohol intake is combined with a fatty food diet.

Fatty liver by itself is a reversible condition if alcohol intake is stopped. However, it can lead to further liver damage if the situation is left uncorrected.

2. Cirrhosis of the Liver:

Once the fatty liver stage is reached and if alcohol intake is continued, cirrhosis of the liver may occur. This is characterized by diffuse liver cell damage and the formation of non-functional fibrous (scar-like) tissue. There is a loss of liver function due to the damage and if the loss becomes great enough, death can occur. Patients with severe cirrhosis also have a 30% risk of developing cancer of the liver in contrast to a less than 5% risk in patients with mild to moderate cirrhosis.

It has been recognized that many chronic alcohol users have normal livers in spite of prolonged alcoholic intake. The reasons for this are not known but may be related to nutrition, constitutional differences, or genetic differences in the alcohol metabolizing enzymes.

PANCREAS

About 40% of all people with pancreatitis (inflammation of the pancreas) are chronic alcohol dependent. Acute pancreatitis is associated with severe abdominal pain and the patient may go into shock. Chronic pancreatitis is also common with alcohol dependent persons, but here, not only is there abdominal pain, but improper food absorption may occur since the pancreas releases enzymes to aid in the digestion and absorption of food. How alcohol causes pancreatitis is unclear, but may be due to the fact that alcohol might stimulate the release of the digestive enzymes from the pancreas and if these enzymes remain in the pancreas, they could start "digesting" the pancreas itself.

MUSCLE

Alcohol is known to cause damage to muscle tissue. In binge drinkers acute muscle damage might occur so, that on "the morning after," there may be some pain and weakness, especially in the limbs. The involved muscles may later become swollen and bruised appearing, indicating a certain degree of muscle tissue death. The dead muscle tissue floating in the blood stream can "clog-up" the kidney's filtration system. If this problem is severe, death could occur from kidney failure.

Chronic alcohol use can also cause peripheral muscle weakness and wasting. This can be due to direct damage by alcohol to the muscle itself or damage to the nerves that control the muscles.

CARDIOVASCULAR SYSTEM

1. The Heart

If an alcohol user becomes deficient in vitamin B1, as can happen due to alcohol's interference with B1 absorption from the small intestine, heart damage can occur. This damage is correctable to a certain point by administration of B1 supplements and cessation of alcohol intake.

Alcohol itself can also cause direct damage to the heart muscle. Alcohol can cause arrhythmias (where the heart does not keep a regular rhythm). This may be due to a decrease in potassium in the body which is caused indirectly by alcohol or may be a direct effect of the acetaldehyde metabolite.

2. Blood Vessel System

Alcohol in moderate amounts causes dilation of blood vessels — especially the blood vessels in the skin. This causes a sensation of warmth and flushing. However, due to this blood vessel dilation, a lot of body heat is lost and internal temperature will drop. With large amounts of alcohol, the mechanisms which normally regulate body temperature can be suppressed and the temperature drop can be severe.

SKIN

As many as 30 to 50% of all alcohol dependent persons have skin diseases. These result from vitamin deficiences, inability to fight infections or the person may neglect to care for abrasions and cuts when they become infected.

If an alcohol user has liver disease, spider angiomas, can be seen, especially in the upper chest area. Acne rosacea, the red nose of alcoholics, may result from chronic blood vessel dilation. Rhinophyma or "brandy nose" is a painless increase in nasal sweat glands which causes an increase in the size of the lower part of the nose.

BLOOD

The most common blood disorder found in alcoholics is an increase in MCV (mean corpuscular volume), which means the red blood cells are larger in size than normal. This blood test is frequently used to check for alcoholism. Even with an adequate intake, alcohol dependent persons can become deficient in folic acid since alcohol decreases the absorption of folic acid from the small intestine. This can lead to a folic acid deficiency anemia. Other blood abnormalities can also occur in chronic alcohol users who receive adequate nutrition, but these can be corrected with alcohol abstinence. Chronic alcohol ingestion can decrease white blood cell (WBC) production with a resultant increase in the number of infections since WBC's are an important part of our body defense system. Also, chronic alcohol intake can decrease platelet function in the body by interfering with the ability of platelets to stick together. Platelets are an important part of the blood clotting mechanism, and this effect of alcohol allows a person to bleed more easily.

RENAL (KIDNEY)

1. Diuresis

Alcohol seems to cause one to urinate more (<u>diuresis</u>) by inhibiting the release of anti-diuretic hormone. This is a compound in the body that normally controls fluid loss from the body. The inhibition of the anti-diuretic hormone results in increased fluid loss and this only occurs when alcohol blood levels are rising, but not when they are stationary or falling. With chronic use, however, alcohol itself may have an anti-diuretic effect and an alcoholic may begin to retain water.

The initial water loss caused by alcohol can also cause the loss of some important body chemcials such as potassium, magnesium, and phosphorus. This could have serious muscle, nerve, and other effects and may be associated with some of the damage seen in the body caused by alcohol.

2. Gout

As was discussed before, the metabolism of alcohol causes an increase in the amount of NADH. With excessive NADH production the body produces lactic acid as a byproduct of converting NADH back to NAD.

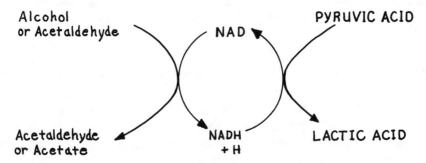

If too much lactic acid is formed, it can cause all sorts of problems by creating an acid environment in the body cells and blood. Lactic acid is not toxic itself, when present in ordinary quantities. However, when present in high quantities, it is like an environmental pollutant.

Another problem with increased lactic acid in the body is that it prevents the secretion of uric acid into the urine. When there is too much uric acid in the blood, it precipitates out as crystals in the joints, which causes swelling and pain.

SEXUAL FUNCTION

There are many popular misconceptions concerning alcohol and sexual function. Most people believe that alcohol acts as an aphrodisiac, and it apparently does increase sexual desire to a certain extent. This is probably due to the loss in inhibition and restraint. The problem lies, however, with the fact that although the desire exists, sexual performance and capabilities are diminished. Little clinical research has been done in this area, but there does seem to be a direct correlation between increasing alcohol blood levels and decreasing sexual performance. The exact mechanism of this action is not known at this time, but the sex hormones may be involved. It is known, however, that many male alcohol dependents often suffer from sexual dysfunction.

Alcohol also affects sexual function in women. Although the mechanim is poorly understood, it appears that in alcoholic women, there may be failure to ovulate.

SUMMARY (Pharmacology of alcohol):

—The RAS- is the portion of the brain which controls "wakefulness" and is affected by alcohol.
—The blood alcohol level- relates to certain behavior. As the blood level rises, a person stumbles, their speech becomes slurred, and eventually they will fall asleep. In many states a level of 0.1, or 100 mg% means a person is legally intoxicated, no matter how sober they may act.
—The CNS effects of chronic alcohol use include:
  —Wernicke-Korsakoff's syndrome, which are severe neurological effects of chronic alcohol exposure, due in part to vitamin B1 deficiency.
  —Confabulation, which is the contriving of stories to fill in gaps in memory.
  —Alcohol dementia, which is the disturbances in memory and thought experienced in many persons during alcohol withdrawal.
—The gastronintestinal effects- include ulceration, blood loss, and both diarrhea and constipation.
—The liver effects of chronic alcohol intake- are fatty liver, and eventually cirrhosis. Also, there is an increased likelihood of liver cancer.
—Pancreatic effects- include pancreatitis.
—Muscle- weakness, swelling, and wasting are commonly seen effects.

—Cardiovascular effects of alcohol- include damage to the heart muscle, and dilation of blood vessels in the skin.
—Skin diseases- are common in alcohol dependent persons.
—Blood cells- (both red and white) and platelets are affected in various ways.
—Kidney- effects of alcohol include diuresis and gout.
—Sexual dysfunction- in both males and females results from chronic alcohol intake.

4. ALCOHOL WITHDRAWAL

Detoxification, or withdrawal from alcohol occurs with decrease in or cessation of alcohol intake. The degree of withdrawal symptoms which occur will depend on: 1) regularity of alcohol use, 2) the time period during which the person has been heavily drinking, and 3) the general physical health of the person.

The symptoms of withdrawal include tremor, perspiring, sleeplessness, restlessness, and a mild increase in blood pressure, pulse rate, respiration and temperature. These symptoms usually begin somewhere between 3 and 10 hours after the last drink and usually subside in 2 to 5 days.

In a chronic drinker with high alcohol intake or one who is in poor physical condition, the minor symptoms may progress to and overlap with "major" withdrawal symptoms. Blood pressure, pulse rate, respiration and temperature may be greatly increased. If a person goes into major withdrawal, they should be kept under strict medical supervision in an intensive care unit-like setting since death can occur due to convulsions or other life-threatening complications. Major withdrawal symptoms usually will subside in three to six days.

SUMMARY (Alcohol withdrawal):

—Alcohol withdrawal symptoms- usually begin 3 to 10 hours after the last drink, and ordinarily subside in 2 to 5 days.

Withdrawal from alcohol is often complicated because most people younger than 40 years old use other psychoactive drugs and may have symptoms which interfere with a textbook description. Simply, alcohol-like sleeping pills, tranquilizers, pain pills, and marijuana are downers, so when a patient undergoes withdrawal they seem quite "up". They appear anxious, nervous, shakey, perspiring, restless, and quite tempermental.

Occasionally a person will be seen who goes through alcohol withdrawal and gets better and then goes through the same symptoms all over again. This may be because the patient forgot to mention they were taking Valium® (or some other tranquilizer) for their nerves. Remember that if patients are dependent on alcohol and other drugs, they will always undergo alcohol withdrawal first because alcohol has a shorter half-life.

CHAPTER TWO-B:

BARBITURATES

1. INTRODUCTION

Since the formation of barbituric acid in 1864 by J.F.W. Adolph von Baeyer, more than 2500 barbiturates have been synthesized, and about 50 compounds marketed. These compounds have been researched and developed for their tranquilizing and sleep inducing effects.

The uses of the barbiturates include:
1. Hypnosis (sleep)
2. Sedation (relaxation)
3. Pre-anesthesia
4. Anesthesia (unconsiousness induced for surgical purposes eg. Pentothal®)
5. Narcoanalysis ("truth serum")
6. Anticonvulsant (anti-seizure eg. phenobarbital)

Some of the more commonly used barbiturates are included in the following table.

GENERIC NAME	TRADE NAME	STREET NAME
Thiopental	Sodium Pentothal®	
Amobarbital	Amytal®	
Pentobarbital	Nembutal®	Yellow Jackets
Secobarbital	Seconal®	Reds
Amobarbital+Secobarb.	Tuinal®	Rainbows
Butabarbital	Butisol®	
Phenobarbital	Luminal®	

2. BIOPHARMACEUTICS
ABSORPTION

The most common route of administration for the barbiturates is oral. The barbiturates are un-ionized (that means they are less water soluble, and more fat soluble) in the stomach and are readily absorbed. Although the presence of food in the stomach may slow absorption, total absorption will still be the same with or without food.

Generally speaking, one of the main determinants of barbiturate absorption is the lipid solubility of the compound. As lipid solubility increases, there is faster absorption, faster entry into the brain tissue, faster metabolism and therefore a shorter duration of action. Based on the duration of action, the barbiturates have been divided into ultra-short, short to moderate, and long-acting classes. These classes are developed mainly from animal studies and human correlation is not exact, however, this classification is still widely used.

DISTRIBUTION

The distribution of a barbiturate and its entry into brain tissue is determined by its lipid solubility (ability to pass through "fatty" membranes). Thiopental is highly lipid soluble and crosses the blood brain barrier (BBB) rapidly. Its sleep inducing and anesthetic effects can be seen rapidly. However, phenobarbital is only slightly lipid soluble and crosses the BBB much more slowly. Even after IV injection, there is at least a 15 minute delay before adequate brain concentrations of phenobarbital are reached to cause sleep.

In general, organs with the greatest blood flow such as the liver, lungs, and kidney, take up the barbiturates first. Then the drug is redistributed to fat tissue in the body. This is one reason why thiopental has such a short duration of CNS action: due to its high lipid solubility, it is rapidly redistributed from brain tissue to more "fatty" areas. Thus, if little or no drug is left in the brain, little CNS action will be seen.

Another barrier, besides the blood brain barrier, which the barbiturates cross is the placental barrier. The placenta is a thick protective membrane which lines the uterus during pregnancy. The more lipid soluble the barbiturate, the more rapidly it crosses the placental barrier. Fetal dependency can result from chronic barbiturate intake by the mother. Also, if barbiturate are taken close to the time of birth, the baby will be born with depressed respirations which can be quite dangerous since a newborn baby lacks the enzymes needed to rid its body of the drug and the respiratory depression may be prolonged.

METABOLISM

With the metabolism of the barbiturates, the body is trying to convert the drug to a less fat soluble, (more water soluble) compound. If the drug is too fat soluble, it will be reabsorbed from the fat lined kidney tubules and re-enter the blood circulation instead of continuing out via urine. The less lipid soluble a barbiturate is, the less metabolism it will require before it can be excreted. For instance, as much as 50% of a dose of phenobarbital is excreted unchanged. Barbital, the least fat soluble of all barbiturates, is excreted almost totally unchanged.

The primary site of barbiturate metabolism is the liver and, as with any other liver metabolized drug, care must be taken when barbiturates are given to persons with liver impairment since they may have a harder time ridding the body of the drug. The liver enzymes which metabolize barbiturates require NADPH, the same energy cofactor used in the MEOS which helps to detoxify alcohol.

BARBITURATE METABOLISM
AND ENZYME INDUCTION

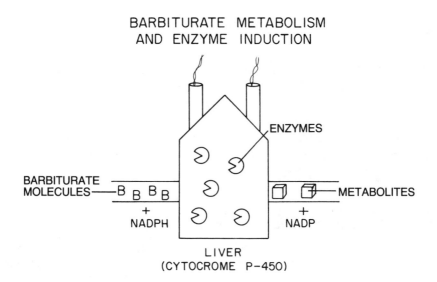

The breakdown products of barbiturates are generally inactive and are excreted in the urine.

Barbiturates can cause the number of their metabolizing enzymes to increase (just as alcohol does). This enzyme induction will cause the metabolism of the barbiturates to proceed at a faster rate, since there will be more enzymes around to perform the metabolism. The increased metabolism with continuous usage of barbiturates accounts in part for the tolerance that is observed to their effects. Enzyme induction can also cause drug interactions to occur since other drugs use these same enzymes for their metabolism.

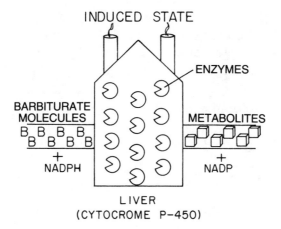

INDUCED STATE

ENZYMES

BARBITURATE
MOLECULES

METABOLITES

B B B B B
B B B B

+
NADPH

+
NADP

LIVER
(CYTOCROME P-450)

EXCRETION

The barbiturates and their metabolites are excreted primarily through the urine. As mentioned before, the more lipid soluble barbiturates can be reabsorbed from the fat-lined kidney tubules and re-enter the blood stream. The only way this recycling can be stopped is by metabolism of the drug to break down products which are more water soluble. The water soluble metabolites cannot re-cross through the fatty barrier of the kidney tubule wall into the blood stream and therefore they will be passed in the urine.

SUMMARY (Biopharmaceutics of barbiturates):

—Absorption- of oral barbiturates depends mainly upon lipid solubility.
—Barbiturates are distributed- to areas with high blood flow first, then redistributed to lipid tissue.
—The barbiturates are metabolized- to inactive compounds usually, and excreted in urine.

3. PHARMACOLOGY

The barbiturates reversibly depress cellular functions, but not all tissues are affected at the same dose. The central nervous system (CNS) is extremely sensitive; so that at doses where sedation or sleep occurs, very little effects are seen on skeletal muscles, the heart, or smooth muscles such as blood vessels and the intestines. Within the brain, the most sensitive area seems to be the reticular activating system (RAS), just as it is with alcohol. In fact, intoxication with barbiturates would appear to an observer to be the same as intoxication with alcohol.

Also, like alcohol, the barbiturates cause a disruption in the normal sleep cycle. With normal sleep, about 20% of sleep time is spent in rapid eye movement (REM) or "dream" sleep. With initial use of barbiturates REM sleep is decreased to only about 10-15%, but this level will eventually climb back to normal with chronic usage. Upon withdrawal from the drug, there is what is known as "REM rebound", where REM sleep could go as high as 100% and nightmares and troubled dreams occur.

Although the drowsiness caused by barbiturates may last only a few hours, distortions in mood and impairment to judgment and fine muscular coordination may persist for 10 to 22 hours after a single dose of barbiturate. This may be due to the presence of some active metabolite, or may be an effect of REM sleep supression.

As the dosage of barbiturate increases, brief periods of brain inactivity (measured by EEG) can occur. With exteme overdoses, all electrical activity of the brain will temporarily cease. This is very important for emergency room workers to know, because a head injury case could appear dead due to a flat EEG, but this could instead be due to a very high barbiturate level.

The barbiturates, like alcohol, have another important effect on the brain in that they raise the seizure threshold — that is, they decrease the sensitivity of the brain to inappropriate electrical discharges, making the brain less susceptible to seizuring. This makes the barbiturates useful in the management of seizure disorder.

SEIZURE THRESHOLD

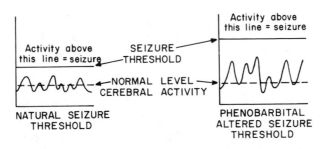

NATURAL SEIZURE THRESHOLD

PHENOBARBITAL ALTERED SEIZURE THRESHOLD

Phenobarbital is especially useful in a type of seizure disorder called grand mal, but this property is not shared by most of the other barbiturates. The anticonvulsant effect is not related to sedation since non-sedating doses are often effective. Since all of the sedative hypnotic drugs make it more difficult to reach the seizure threshold, withdrawal from barbiturates causes a rebound or increased chance of having a seizure. It is because of this fact that convulsions can occur during barbiturate withdrawal even in persons who are not normally seizure prone. This is especially seen in chronic barbiturate dependent people.

The barbiturates, like all sedative hypnotic drugs, can also cause tolerance. Acute tolerance can occur after a single dose, but this only lasts about 48 hours. Chronic tolerance occurs with repeated usage and is due to two mechanisms. The first mechanism is enzyme duplication. This means that the drug is being broken down faster than it was when taken the first time due to the presence of more metabolizing enzymes. Thus, the duration of action would be shorter. However, this mechanism alone does not completely explain tolerance since a certain blood level of barbiturate will not cause the same reactions in a chronic user as in a naive user. Therefore, a second mechanism of tolerance must exist in the CNS, but the details of its action are not yet fully understood. It is known, however, that somehow the brain must establish other ways to deal with a constant exposure to the drug.

The time required to develop chronic tolerance is dependent on the dose of barbiturate. The lower the daily dose, the longer the time required to develop tolerance. A cross tolerance to other sedative-hypnotics also occurs as tolerance develops towards the barbiturates. There can also be a marked variation in the degree of tolerance between different people and even with a single person on different days. The factors responsible for the variability are not known, but diet, emotional excitement and drug interactions may be responsible. Despite the variability, there is a definite maximum dose of barbiturate which can be tolerated and exceeding that dose by even a small amount (for instance, 100mg added to 1000mg or 2000mg) can produce a marked degree of intoxication.

A very serious aspect of barbiturate tolerance is that the fatal dose may rise initially as tolerance develops but it has a definite limit. As a person becomes tolerant, they tend to increase the barbiturate dose so the same effect can always be felt. As they are doing this, they come closer and closer to the lethal level and eventually there is only a narrow margin between the dose where effects are felt and the dose where death occurs.

THERAPEUTIC INDEX

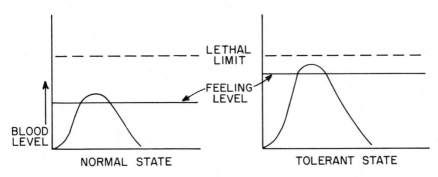

*Note also that large amounts of drug may be present to affect body systems and cause drug interaction even when patient feels little.

Death from barbiturate overdose occurs due to respiratory arrest. Normal automatic respiration is controlled by three centers — two in the brain and one which is mediated by oxygen detectors located in the carotid arteries of the neck and in the main artery from the heart. The two centers in the brain are the first to be affected by the depressant action of the drug. Eventually, with progressively higher blood levels, all the stimuli to breathe are depressed and respiration ceases. Since a continuous oxygen supply is needed to maintain cellular life, cellular death occurs. Brain tissue is the most sensitive to oxygen deprivation and it is the first to die, so even if respiration is artificially restored before total body death occurs, at least some degree of brain damage will probably result.

SUMMARY (Pharmacology of barbiturates):

—REM rebound- along with nightmares occurs upon withdrawal.
—Seizure threshold- is raised, and the barbiturates are used in the treatment of some seizure disorders.
—Tolerance and cross tolerance- with other sedative hypnotic drugs occurs.
—Overdose- results in respiratory arrest.

4. ADVERSE REACTIONS

WITHDRAWAL
Withdrawal can occur from prolonged usage of high daily doses. Withdrawal can be extremely dangerous and death can result. The

withdrawal symptoms are almost identical to those seen with alcohol. However, the onset and duration of the withdrawal may vary depending on the type of barbiturate used (i.e. the onset of symptoms will be sooner with the shorter acting barbiturates and the length of exposure shorter). Another very important difference between alcohol and barbiturate withdrawal is that a person may suddenly experience "major" symptoms such as life threatening convulsions without the previous presence of any minor withdrawal signs. Thus barbiturate withdrawal should be carefully monitored in a hospital setting since major withdrawal could have an extremely abrupt onset and seems to appear without any minor withdrawal symptoms.

IDIOSYNCRATIC EXCITATION
Certain people, especially the very young (under 10 years) and the very old (older than 65 years), may experience a paradoxical excitation effect with usage of a barbiturate. The effect will appear almost the same as if some sort of stimulant had been taken. The exact mechanism of this reaction is unknown, but may be due to some fundamental physiological or chemical difference in these people.

HANGOVER
"Hangover" can occur with the barbiturates even from relatively small hypnotic doses. This effect is seen especially with the longer acting barbiturates, such as phenobarbital. After the initial period of sedation has passed, listlessness, nausea, vomiting, and dizziness may occur and emotional disturbances may be accentuated. The exact mechanism of this effect is not known.

INTRAVENOUS USE
Some barbiturate abusers inject the contents of capsules or tablets into their veins so that blood levels of the barbiturate will have a high, rapid peak. This is done to obtain a "rush" (a rapid high). The barbiturates are alkaline compounds which are highly irritating to the blood vessels. If the drug is accidentally injected into an artery, the artery will spasm and it can collapse. If this happens, for instance in the arm, the loss of blood supply could result in permanent damage to the hand and fingers so that amputation may be necessary. Injecting under the skin is also quite harmful and a person coming to the emergency room under these conditions will have a great deal of inflammation, pain, and swelling in the affected body area.

BIRTH DEFECTS

Thus far, birth defects caused by barbiturates have been seen only in animal studies. Further testing needs to be done to determine the effect on human embryonic development.

SUMMARY (Adverse reactions):

—Withdrawal symptoms- are almost identical to those seen with alcohol.
—I.V. use of barbiturates- gives a rapid high, but can result in damage to the blood vessel and surrounding tissues.

5. DRUG INTERACTIONS

DUE TO ENZYME INDUCTION

Chronic barbiturate use causes an increase in liver enzyme activity (enzyme induction). Since there are other drugs which use these same ·enzymes for their metabolism, drug interactions can occur due to this mechanism. Since the other drugs are metabolized much more quickly than normal, their desired therapeutic effect will be decreased. It may then be necessary to increase the dose of these particular drugs. However, if the barbiturate is subsequently discontinued, the enzyme induction will stop and the number of enzymes will drop back to normal. It will then be necessary to decrease the dose of these other drugs accordingly to avoid an overdose situation. Some examples of drugs which react in this way are:

> warfarin (Coumadin®)
> chlorpromazine (Thorazine®)
> steroids such as hydrocortisone, dexamethasone
> tricyclic antidepressants, such as amitryptyline
>   (Elavil®) and imipramine (Tofranil®)

DUE TO INCREASED CNS DEPRESSION

As described earlier, increased central nervous system depression is seen when barbiturates are used with other sedative hypnotic drugs. It is also usually seen in combination with antihistamines (drugs like Benadryl®), narcotic analgesics (drugs like morphine) and some antipsychotic drugs (such as Thorazine®).

SUMMARY (Drug interactions):

—Due to enzyme induction- with several drugs.
—Due to increased CNS depression- with many classes of drugs.

CHAPTER TWO-C:

BENZODIAZEPINES

1. INTRODUCTION

The benzodiazepines have been marketed in the U.S. for only about twenty-five years. Today, and for the past several years, they have been the most frequently prescribed class of drugs. At the time of this writing there were 12 members of this class marketed in the U.S., although over 2000 types of benzodiazepine have been synthesized. Following is a table listing approximate half-lives and peaks of activity of the benzodiazepines.

GENERIC NAME	TRADE NAME	HALF-LIFE (HOURS)	PEAK EFFECT	ACTIVE METABOLITES
diazepam	Valium®	20-50	1-2	yes
chlordiazepoxide	Librium®	5-30	2-4	yes-many
clorazepate	Tranxene®	—	—	yes
prazepam	Centrax/Verstran®	—	6	yes
flurazepam	Dalmane®	—	—	yes
halazepam	Paxipam®	7	1.3	yes
oxazepam	Serax®	5-10	1-2	none
alprazolam	Xanax®	12-19	0.7-1.6	yes
temazepam	Restoril®	9-12	2-3	insignificant
triazolam	Halcion®	2.3	0.5-1.5	yes
clonazepam	Clonipin®	20-40	1-2	yes
lorazepam	Ativan®	10-20	2	none

Clinical structures, along with more specific information about the active metabolites are located in the appendix.

The clinical uses of the benzodiazepines are:
1. anxiety (all members of class)
2. sleep (usually flurazepam or temazepam, but other too)
3. pre-anesthesia (diazepam)
4. pre-obstetrics (diazepam)
5. muscle relaxation (diazepam)
6. seizures (diazepam, clonazepam, clorazepate)

The importance of the benzodiazepines is that they mimic already existing substances that help calm the brain. Even though the exact mechanism is not yet known it seems that some people who have a decrease in the naturally occurring "releasers" and these persons may need an extra boost. There may be other ways of increasing these brain substances, such as excercise or diet. The use of tranquilizers for conditions for greater than three months on a daily basis is becoming less acceptable and recently physicians have been discouraged from prescribing benzodiazepines tranquilizers for the anxieties of everyday living.

2. BIOPHARMACEUTICS

ABSORPTION

The benzodiazepines are basically lipid soluble compounds and are easily absorbed from the gastrointestinal tract. Peak blood levels of the drugs usually occur at about two to four hours after an oral dose. Chlorazepate has a small quirk in that it requires a high level of acidity in the stomach for complete absorption. For this reason, it is often avoided in people who take antacids regularly or any drug which decreases the production of stomach acid, and in elderly people since they often have a decreased production of stomach acid.

DISTRIBUTION

Since the benzodiazepines are lipid soluble, they can easily cross the blood brain barrier. They can also cross the placental barrier quite rapidly, and may cause withdrawal signs and symptoms in newborn children. If these drugs are taken in early pregnancy, birth defects may result. Also, if these drugs are given just prior to delivery, prolonged sedation in the newborn may result. This is due to the fact that a newborn baby has low levels of drug metabolizing enzymes, therefore a prolonged action is seen. Benzodiazepines are not recommended for use in mothers who are breast feeding. Peak metabolite levels in milk may occur as late as 2 days after the dose, so predicting the peak time after a dose is impossible. Small infants are unable to eliminate benzodiazepines efficiently, as mentioned above, and again the drug will accumulate.

METABOLISM

Most of the metabolites of the benzodiazepines are also active drugs. The benzodiazepines which have metabolites have a longer overall drug effect. Their metabolism is primarily carried out in the liver and since there are so many active metabolites, accumulation can occur in people with impaired liver function (such as those with liver disease or the very old) just as it does in infants. Lorazepam, oxazepam, and temazepam have no active metabolites (see previous table), and require only addition of a water soluble glucuronic acid molecule to be excreted. As would be expected, they would have a shorter duration of action. These benzodiazepines would probably be the drugs of choice for people with any type of liver impairment. An interesting aside to the metabolism of the benzodiazepines is that a cigarette smoker requires higher doses of these drugs to relieve anxiety than do non-smokers. It is believed that mechanism of this action is that cigarette smoking causes the benzodiazepines to use an alternative metabolic pathway which significantly decreases the number of active metabolites of the benzodiazepines and thereby causes a decreased effect.

EXCRETION

After metabolism and changing to water soluble substances, the benzodiazepines are excreted via the urine.

3. PHARMACOLOGY

The pharmacology of the benzodiazepines is basically similar to that of all sedative hypnotics. The benzodiazepines have a slightly different mechanism of action in the reticular activating system (RAS) than does alcohol, however. Alcohol causes the release of dopamine in the RAS and dopamine causes stimulation of the depressant side of the RAS. (Review figure 13.) The benzodiazepines, on the other hand, cause a release of GABA (gama-amino-butyric acid) in the RAS. GABA is a depressor of the stimulation side of the reticular activating system, so again the depressant side dominates.

The benzodiazepines also seem to act in a part of the brain called the limbic system which is a section of the brain involved with emotions. It is believed that benzodiazepines produce an anti-anxiety effect in the limbic system, however, the exact mechanism of this effect is unknown.

Several of the benzodiazepines are useful as sleep inducing agents (hypnotics). The benzodiazepines, unlike other hypnotic agents, cause little or no REM sleep suppression with usage or REM rebound upon withdrawal. Tolerance to their action is also much slower in developing than to the barbiturates and other hypnotics. Diazepam (Valium®) has also been found to have useful muscle-relaxant properties that the other benzodiazepines lack. Unfortunately, the muscle relaxant dose is well into the sedation range so sedation is a definite side effect. Also, diazepam (and some other benzodiazepines) raise the seizure threshold for epileptic attacks and is especially useful in the condition known as status epilepticus where seizure activity is continuous without stopping. (Review figure 17.) In this situation, diazepam is administered intravenously. Diazepam can also be used for the seizure activity seen in severe sedative hypnotic withdrawals.

The benzodiazepines have a very high therapeutic/lethal ratio, which allows for a greater margin of safety. This means that the lehal level is very much greater than doses regularly used in therapeutic situations, such as for sleep, tranquilization, epilepsy, etc. With the usual oral doses heart, circulatory, or respiratory problems are uncommon.

4. ADVERSE REACTIONS
   a. Sedation.
   b. Slurred speech.
   c. Dizziness.
   d. Obesity.
   e. Decreased muscle tone.
   f. Paradoxical excitation: just like the barbiturates, the benzodiazepines can cause a stimulant like effect in some people, especially the very young and the elderly. The exact mechanism for this reaction is unknown.
   g. Tolerance.
   h. Physical dependence: like all sedative hypnotics, physical dependence to the benzodiazepines can occur. The withdrawal is usually quite mild, characterized by some sleep disturbance and anxiety. Due to the long half-life of most benzodiazepines, signs of withdrawals do not appear until 3 to 7 days after cessation and last for 1 to 3 weeks. Deaths during withdrawal have been known to occur, however, this was when the daily amounts used were extremely high.

   There is probably a low dose and high dose withdrawal syndrome. The former is similar to minor withdrawal syndrome of alcohol but there seems to be more emotional disturbance. In the high dose withdrawal syndrome frank psychoptic behavior and seizures have been reported.

SUMMARY:

BIOPHARMACEUTICS: The benzodiazepines are lipid soluble compounds which are well absorbed from the gastrointestinal tract and distributed throughout the fatty areas of the body. Many benzodiazepines have active metabolites which prolong their effects.

PHARMACOLOGY: The benzodiazepines act on the RAS, but in by slightly different mechanism than does alcohol.

REM sleep appears to be little affected by benzodiazepines.

OTHER SEDATIVE-HYPNOTICS

The following table lists generic and trade names, and half-lives of some other important sedative-hypnotic drugs which will be disussed in this section.

GENERIC NAME	TRADE NAMES	NORMAL HALF-LIFE (HOURS)
meprobamate	Equanil®, Miltown®	10
methyprylon	Noludar®	4
glutethimide	Doriden®	5-22
ethclorvynol	Placidyl®	5-6
chloral hydrate	Noctec®	8
methazualone	Quaalude®, Parest®	biphasic 2-3 & 18-24

Although these drugs are prescribed less often than barbiturates and benzodiazepines, they are still seen in many overdose cases. These overdoses are mainly in older people who have been prescribed these drugs for years for sleep or relaxation, who are labeled as drug dependent and who certainly require a different approach than heroin cocaine dependent persons. Since most of these people are elderly (over 55 years old) there are frequent complaints during withdrawal.

1. MEPROBAMATE

BIOPHARMACEUTICS

Meprobamate is well absorbed from the gastrointestinal tract with peak effect in 2 to 3 hours. Meprobamate is about 90% metabolized in the liver with about 10% excreted unchanged in the urine. During metabolism, the liver usually adds an -OH group (hydroxylation) and then adds a glucuronide molecule (conjugation) to make the compound more water soluble. Chronic use of meprobamate can lead to replication of the microsomal enzyme system and thus speed up its own metabolism. Since other sedative-hypnotic drugs such as the barbiturates, use this enzyme pathway, too, there is increased metabolism and subsequent decrease in half-life of these drugs as well. This results in them having less of an effect.

PHARMACOLOGY

The exact mechanism of action of meprobamate is unknown. Meprobamate has muscle relaxant properties and raises the CNS seizure threshold, as well as causing sedation and sleep. Like the other SHDs, meprobamate causes a REM sleep surpression so that REM rebound will occur with withdrawal. Tolerance to meprobamate does occur and cross tolerance also exists with barbiturates and alcohol. This means that a person tolerant to meprobamate may also be tolerant to the effects of other sedative-hypnotic drugs so that high doses of those drugs would be needed to cause an effect. It also means that other sedative hypnotic drugs such as the barbiturates can be substituted to depress withdrawal from meprobamate.

Sudden withdrawal from high doses (usually greater than 2gm a day which equals five 400mg tablets) of meprobamate may result in muscular twitching and even convulsions. The withdrawal syndrome usually occurs within 36 to 48 hours after cessation of drug and shows the characteristic withdrawal syndrome of barbiturates. If seizures or other major withdrawal symptoms do occur, they usually occur 24 to 48 hours after the last dose. Severe withdrawal signs and symptoms are usually only seen in persons taking 3 grams or more a day (more than seven 400mg tablets daily), for at least 6 months.

As with most other psychoactive drugs, meprobamate crosses the placental barrier, and also goes into breast milk. It should not be used during pregnancy or by mothers who are breast feeding.

SUMMARY:

—Biopharmaceutics- Chronic use causes enzyme induction.

—Pharmacology- Withdrawal can lead to muscle twitching and occasionally seizures.

2. METHYPRYLON

BIOPHARMACEUTICS

Methyprylon is chemically similar to the barbiturates. However, methyprylon is less lipid soluble than the barbiturates and the extent of its absorption is really not known. The half-life is approximately 4 hours. Ninety-seven percent of the absorbed drug is metabolized in the liver and this is mostly done by hydroxylation and conjugation. The main route of excretion is through the urine. Chronic methyprylon usage has been shown to induce the liver microsomal enzyme systems. Therefore, a cross tolerance to other sedative hypnotic drugs would be expected.

PHARMACOLOGY

Tolerance, physical dependence and psychological dependence can occur with chronic use of methyprylon. The withdrawal syndrome is characterized by insomnia, confusion, agitation, hallucinations and possible convulsions as is seen with the barbiturates and other sedative-hypnotic drugs. It usually begins within 24 hours after cessation of the drug.

SUMMARY:

—Biopharmaceutics- chronic use results in enzyme induction.

—Pharmacology- Effects and withdrawal are basically the same as barbiturates and other sedative-hypnotics.

3. GLUTETHIMIDE

BIOPHARMACEUTICS

Glutethimide is also structurally related to the barbiturates, but it is much more lipid soluble than methyprylon, therefore its absorption and lipid distribution is greater. The drug is metabolized to a great extent by the liver into several active compounds and at least one of the metabolites has CNS depressant activity of its own. Many of the breakdown products enter what is known as the <u>enterohepatic</u> <u>circulation</u> where the compounds are secreted into the intestines through the bile and then re-absorbed from the bowel back into the blood stream. This leads to alternating drowsiness and wakefulness. Thus, their excretion in the urine is quite slow. The half-life is any where from 5 to 22 hours. Glutethimide may also cause liver microsomal enzyme induction and therefore tolerance and cross tolerance exist.

PHARMACOLOGY

Like other sedative-hypnotic drugs, glutethimide suppresses REM sleep and can cause tolerance and dependence characterized by a withdrawal syndrome. There is one thing that distinguishes glutethimide from all other sedative-hypnotics and this is the fact that glutethimide has strong anticholinergic effects. From the introductory chapter, you may recall that the cholinergic nervous system is known as the parasympathetic nervous system (PSNS) and uses acetylcholine as the neurotransmitter. It is basically a depressing or toning down system and it also controls digestion. It is opposed by the sympathetic nervous system (SNS) which causes excitation or stimulation. Glutethimide has anticholinergic activity, which means that it blocks the responses of the PSNS or cholinergic system and allows the SNS to dominate. Therefore, the heart beats faster, the intestines slow down digestion (so that constipation could occur), saliva secretion slows (mouth becomes dry), pupils dilate, sweating stops, and the person may appear agitated even though he has taken a "downer". When sweating stops, the main body-heat removing system is eliminated, so blood vessels in the skin dilate trying to radiate off the normal body heat. Thus, a person who has taken a great quantity of glutethimide would appear flushed (red), with a dry mouth, rapid heart beat, and dilated pupils. With extreme overdose, not only will these signs and symptoms be present, but respiratory depression will occur due to CNS depression as with all sedative-hypnotic drugs. In an acute situation, the half-life may be as long as 105 hours, so that the person's medical management may take several days. Thus even though glutethimide shares in common all the general properties of the sedative-hypnotic drugs, therapeutic and toxicity management is more difficult, because it also has these very distinctive anticholinergic properties as well.

SUMMARY:

—Biopharmaceutics- Metabolized to several active compounds.

—Pharmacology- Can be distinguished from other sedative-hypnotics by strong anticholinergic effects.

4. ETHCHLORVYNOL

BIOPHARMACEUTICS

Ethchlorvynol is rapidly absorbed and its effects can be seen within 15 to 30 minutes following ingestion. Maximal blood levels are reached within 1 to 1½ hours. The duration of action is very short with the half-life being only 5 to 6 hours. Ethchlorvynol is metabolized in the liver and excreted in the urine. At least in animals it does not seem to stimulate the induction of liver enzymes systems, but further studies need to be done with human subjects.

PHARMACOLOGY

Although the effect of REM sleep of ethchlorvynol has not been studied, ethchlorvynol causes tolerance and dependence like other sedative-hypnotic drugs and death occurs in acute overdose due to respiratory failure.

SUMMARY:

—Biopharmaceutics- onset of effects is fairly rapid.

—Pharmacology- basically the same as other sedative hypnotics.

5. CHLORAL HYDRATE

BIOPHARMACEUTICS

Chloral hydrate is rapidly absorbed from the gastrointestinal tract. Chloral hydrate is metabolized by the alcohol dehydrogenase (ADH) enzyme system in the liver to form a metabolite called trichloroethanol, which is also an active sedative-hypnotic drug. The half-life for chloral hydrate and its metabolite, trichloroethanol, is approximately 8 hours. Excretion is mainly through the urine.

PHARMACOLOGY

The mechanism of action of chloral hydrate is not completely known, but the metabolite trichloroethanol seems to be an important component of the action. There are conflicting reports concerning the effect of chloral hydrate on REM sleep and apparently REM rebound does not occur to a significant degree when the drug is withdrawn. The intoxication properties of chloral hydrate appear to be low, but can be greatly increased by simultaneous administration of alcohol. This is because both alcohol and trichloroethanol use the same enzyme (ADH) for metabolism, and can competitively inhibit one another's inactivation. This mixture is what is known as "knockout drops" or "Mickey Finn". Chloral hydrate and alcohol used together may cause dilation of the blood vessels which is characterized by a fast heart beat, palpitations, facial flushing, and a general feeling of uneasiness or dysphoria (the opposite of euphoria).

Another important drug interaction occurs with chloral hydrate and warfarin (Coumadin®), which is a blood thinner. Many types of drugs are bound to protein molecules which are part of the blood. These proteins are called <u>plasma proteins</u>. When a drug is bound to a plasma protein like this, it is inactive; that is to say, it is free to bind with a receptor site and cause an action in the cell. When taken alone, one drug's plasma protein binding is not significant. However, when these two drugs are taken together, each of which have a high degree of plasma protein binding, they compete for binding sites and one of the two drugs will be displaced. When drug molecules are displaced from this binding site, they become free to bind to their cellular receptor sites and cause an action. If many drug molecules are suddenly displaced from plasma protein binding and bind to receptor sites, an intense drug reaction can occur with even a possibility of an overdose. The trichloroethanol molecules can displace Coumadin® from its plasma protein binding sites and too much blood thinning can occur. This makes a person much more susceptible to bleeding and many problems can occur.

Like the other sedative-hypnotics, chloral hydrate can cause tolerance and physical dependence, and the withdrawal syndrome is similar to that for barbiturates, though less intense.

SUMMARY:

—Biopharmaceutics- Metabolized to another active sedative-hypnotic drug, trichloroethanol.

—Pharmacology- A potent synergistic effect occurs with alcohol.

6. METHAQUALONE

BIOPHARMACEUTICS

In man, 99% of a dose of methaqualone is absorbed in 2 hours. This accounts for the feeling of a "rush" which is obtained with methaqualone, since the blood level peak is rapid and high. This undoubtedly is one of the main reasons why methaqualone has become widely abused. Methaqualone is broken down (via hydroxylation) by the liver microsomal enzyme system and excretion (of hydroxylated and conjugated metabolites) occurs mainly through the urine.

Methaqualone binds actively to proteins. Under normal physiologic conditions, and at dosages in the normal range, 90% of the drug is bound to the plasma proteins. This great amount of protein binding results in a half-life described as "<u>biphasic</u>". The over all half-life of methaqualone is from 18 to 42 hours. However, when blood samples are drawn, and tested for free drug in the serum, it appears to the tester that half the drug is gone in just 2 to 3 hours. This is because, after going into the blood, much methaqualone is redistributed from the blood to protein and fatty tissues. This is called the distribution phase. Gradually, as the drug remaining in the plasma is metabolized, methaqualone becomes unbound and returns to the serum where it can circulate to the liver and be metabolized. This phase, which is more gradual, is called the terminal phase, and results in the prolonged half-life.

PHARMACOLOGY

The exact mechanism of the sedative hypnotic effect of methaqualone is unknown and there is also disagreement as to whether REM sleep is affected or not. Since methaqualone is currently such an abused drug, it should always be kept in mind that tolerance and dependence can occur and withdrawal from high doses may precipitate life-threatening convulsions.

Like chloral hydrate, methaqualone may cause displacement of other highly protein bound drugs because of its high percentage of protein binding.

SUMMARY:

—Biopharmaceutics- Very rapid absorption occurs, giving a "rush" effect. A high degree of protein binding is seen, which results in a biphasic half-life.

—Pharmacology- Tolerance, dependence, and withdrawal occur, as with other sedative hypnotic drugs.

CHAPTER 3

Narcotics and
Narcotic Antagonists

CHAPTER THREE

NARCOTICS AND NARCOTIC ANTAGONISTS

HISTORY

The narcotic analgesics are also commonly referred to as opioids. This is because they have actions similar to morphine which is the chief active ingredient in opium. Opium is derived from the opium poppy, Papaver somniferum, which is native to Turkey. (You can't get opium from a California Golden Poppy ... so don't try!) The opium poppy yields several sustances called alkaloids. (An alkaloid is one type of drug which can be extracted from a plant.) These alkaloids include morphine, codeine, and papaverine. Papaverine is a smooth muscle relaxant, and lacks morphine-like effects. Morphine was identified in 1803, and codeine in 1832, however the history of opium use probably pre-dates its mention in ancient Samarian writings of 4000BC. Heroin is an example of a semisynthetic opium derivative. Meperidine (Demerol®) is not derived from an opium alkaloid. It is a synthetic narcotic analgesic, first introduced in the USA in 1939. Methadone and its chemical cousin, propoxyphene (Davon®), are chemically very different from morphine, just as meperidine is, but still have the opioid narcotic analgesic (pain relief) action.

CHEMISTRY

Drugs which cause a certain response in the body to occur are called agonists. Morphine, codeine, heroin, methadone, and meperidine are examples of narcotic agonists. They cause analgesia (loss of sense of pain) in appropriate doses. In addition to discussing agonists in this chapter, narcotic antagonists (drugs which oppose, or block, the action of narcotic agonists will be discussed. Naloxone and naltrexone are examples of narcotic antagonists. There are also drugs which have properties of both agonists and antagonists. They cause analgesia like the agonists, and can block effects of the narcotic agonists like the antagonists. Pentazocine (Talwin®) is an example of an agonist-antagonist (or partial agonist). The properties of the narcotic agonists, antagonists, and agonist-antagonists will be discussed in this chapter.

EPIDEMIOLOGY/CRIME

A 1979 study by the National Institute on Drug Abuse found that 1% of Americans over the age of 12 had used heroin at least once, and 5% had used other narcotic analgesics for non-medical reasons. An estimated 500,000 Americans are opiate dependent. The costs to society are much greater than this implies. In ranking of drug related causes for emergency room visits (1980):

> —Heroin/morphine is number 3 (Alcohol in combination with other drugs is number one, and Valium® is number 2)
> —Propoxyphene (Darvon®) is number 8
> —Methadone is number 17

Narcotic analgesics account for 26.6% of drug-related deaths reported by emergency rooms. In addition to costs in life, and medical care, you may recall the narcotics, especially heroin, are associated with very high crime rates against property (ie. theft, embezzlement, forgery, etc; as opposed to crimes against persons ie. murder, rape, assault).

CHAPTER THREE-A:

NARCOTIC ANALGESICS

Following is a table listing the more commonly used narcotic analgesics, grouped according to chemical similarity, along with their half-lives, and duration of analgesia. (Large quantities of the drug persist in the body long after the analgesia wears off.)

GENERIC NAME	TRADE NAME	HALF-LIFE (hrs)	DURATION (hrs) OF ANALGESIA
morphine		2-3	4-5
codeine		3-4	4-6
heroin		2.5	—
hydromorphone	Dilaudid®	2-4	4-5
oxycodone	Percodan®	4-5	3-4
oxymorphone	Numorphan®	4-5	4-5
hydrocodone	Vicodin®	3-4	4-8
levorphanol	Levo-Dromoran®	—	6-8
meperidine	Demerol®	3-4	2-4
alphaprodine	Nisentyl®	2	1-2
fentanyl	Sublimaze®	5-21min	1-2
methadone	Dolophine®	22-25	3-6
propoxyphene	Darvon®	6-12	—
levo alpha acetylmethadol (LAAM)		—	—
*pentazocine	Talwin®	2-3	2-3
*nalbuphine	Nubain®	5	3-6
*butorphanol	Stadol®	2.5-3.5	3-4

*These drugs have the properties of agonist-antagonist.

The narcotic analgesics, in addition to their main use as analgesics (pain relievers) are used for cough suppression (eg. codeine), and anti-diarrheals.

1. BIOPHARMACEUTICS

ABSORPTION

Morphine and most of the other narcotic compounds are poorly absorbed with oral use. The opiates are basic (or alkaline) so they are <u>ionized</u> (which means they exist in a more water soluble form) in the acidity of the stomach, and therefore, are not absorbed from the stomach. With the basic environment of the intestines, they are no longer ionized, but they can be quickly conjugated, which makes them unavailable for absorption. The drug molecules which are absorbed must first go through the liver before reaching the main blood stream and many molecules will be conjugated in the liver and therefore inactivated. Thus, morphine is erratically absorbed with oral use and the effect is usually 1/3 to 1/5 as potent as with intravenous use.

INACTIVATION OF NARCOTICS IN THE G.I. TRACT

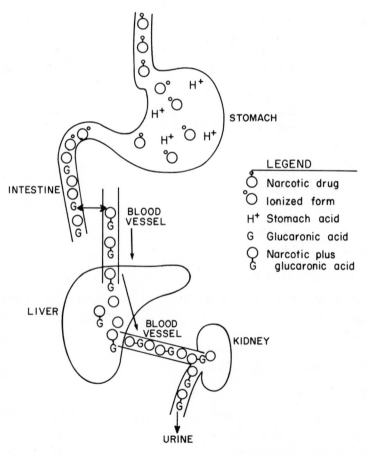

STOMACH

INTESTINE

BLOOD VESSEL

LIVER

BLOOD VESSEL

KIDNEY

URINE

LEGEND

○ Narcotic drug
○ Ionized form
H⁺ Stomach acid
G Glucaronic acid
○ Narcotic plus
G glucaronic acid

The opiates are well absorbed with hypodermic needle use. When narcotics are injected just under the skin (subcutaneously) it is called "skin popping". Intravenous use is called "slamming" or "mainlining". "Snorting" or nasal inhalation is also a common means of using narcotics, especially heroin, since the drug reaches the main blood stream without going through the liver, just as it does with hypodermic needle use. Snorting is usually done by beginners who can then procede to skin popping and finally mainlining for maximal effect.

Some narcotics are at least partially effective orally, because they are not so readily conjugated, and tablet or capsule preparations are made. These preparations include:

1. codeine
2. oxycodone (Percodan®, Percocet®)
3. meperidine (Demerol®)
4. pentazocine (Talwin®)
5. propoxyphene (Darvon®)
6. methadone (Dolophine®)
7. LAAM (an investigational drug)

DISTRIBUTION

The narcotics concentrate in tissues, especially in the kidney, liver, skeletal muscle, lung, and spleen. The precise reasons for this are unclear. These are called "silent receptor sites" since the main effects of the narcotics occur in the central nervous system. Very slowly the drugs will redistribute out of these silent receptor sites.

Only small amounts of narcotics cross through the blood brain barrier (BBB) so that the brain concentration is much less than the concentration in the blood. However, the central nervous system is so sensitive that only minute amounts are needed to cause a pharmacologic effect.

One percent of a dose also crosses the placental barrier so that fetal dependency can occur. Since the fetal metabolizing capabilities are much less developed than an adult's, only very small amounts are necessary to cause dependency. In ordinary doses, only small amounts of the narcotic analgesics are secreted in breast milk, and the effects on an infant appear to be insignificant. However, heroin abuse has been associated with high enough levels to result in newborn addiction, or delay of withdrawal in an addicted newborn.

METABOLISM

The metabolism of narcotic analgesics is more complicated than that of most of the sedative-hypnotic drugs which have been discussed. Their metabolism is summarized here and covered in more detail in the appendix.

Many of the metabolites of the narcotic analgesics are also potent analgesics. The narcotics which have several active metabolites, such as methadone and LAAM, usually have prolonged half-lives.

The final metabolic product of the narcotic analgesics and their metabolites is almost always a water soluble molecule formed by conjugation.

Chronic use of opiates, unlike the sedative hypnotics, does not cause liver microsomal enzyme induction. On the contrary, when liver microsomes are prepared from animals receiving repeated doses of morphine, they show progressively decreasing ability to form the major metabolic products of narcotic analgesics and other drugs which might utilize the same metabolic pathways.

EXCRETION

Excretion of the narcotic drugs is largely through the urine after metabolism to water soluble metabolites. Some excretion also occurs in expired air and bile.

Suprisingly, high concentrations of methadone and its metabolites are excreted into sweat. Usually, a person has a volume of 500ml (around a pint) of sweat per day. However, during periods of strenuous exercise or environmental temperatures of 100°F or more, the volume could go as high as 2400ml (around 2½ quarts) of sweat per day. When the sweat volume is this high, much methadone can be lost and there have been reports of people developing withdrawal signs and symptoms under these conditions.

SUMMARY (Biopharmaceutics)

—Many narcotic analgesics are poorly absorbed on oral use. However, they are well absorbed when given under the skin or when "snorted".

—The central nervous system is very sensitive to the narcotics. Fetal addiction may occur fairly easily.

—Metabolism is very complicated, often with active metabolites. Enzyme induction does not occur, apparently.

—Most narcotic metabolites are excreted as conjugated compounds, in the urine, although there may be significant excreticn in certain cases via other routes.

2. PHARMACOLOGY

MECHANISM OF ACTION

The mechanism of action of narcotics is not known. It is known that there are specific narcotic receptor sites on cell membranes in the brain and other places in the body. The existence of these receptors has been postulated for a long time. However, the reason for the presence of receptors for substances alien to the body was not explored until just recently. It was found that within the body are substances called "enkephalins" which act as the body's own narcotics and are probably involved in the regulation of pain perception, and the emotional response to it. Enkephalins are found in the brain, spinal cord, and in the peripheral nervous system of the body. In addition to regulating pain perception, the enkephalins may play a role in emotionality in general by producing feelings of pleasure just as the opiates produce euphoria. It has even been theorized that people with low levels of enkephalins might be more susceptible to depression. The ancient practice of acupuncture may also be involved with enkephalins since in certain studies, the mechanism of pain relief caused by acupuncture appeared to be due to the release of enkephalins.

It appears then that the narcotic drugs bind with enkephalin receptors in the body and produce the same effects as do the enkephalins themselves. In fact, if high doses of enkephalins are given to laboratory animals, they become "addicted" and a typical narcotic withdrawal syndrome can be caused when these high doses are stopped. It is believed that during times of addiction to either narcotics or high levels of enkephalins, the normal body production of enkephalins is decreased considerably, since they are not needed. When the narcotic administration is stopped, the body goes through a period of readjustment until the body's own enkephalin production returns to normal. This readjustment period is called withdrawal. Thus, the study of use, addiction, and withdrawal of the narcotics is now intimately tied to the study of the body's own narcotic, the enkephalins.

ORGAN SYSTEM EFFECTS

The narcotics, in general, produce a variety of effects on the different organ systems of the body. The effects produced by morphine will be considered the prototype of the whole narcotic class and each organ system will be reviewed individually.

A. Central Nervous System Effects

In general, morphine produces analgesia, drowsiness, changes in mood, and a mental "clouding" or impairment of intellectual processes.

(1) Analgesia

Continuous, dull pain is relieved more effectively than intermittent sharp pain. Morphine may raise the level of pain perception slightly, but the most significant part of its analgesic action is that it reduces the mental distress which can accompany pain. Thus, morphine acts more on what is known as the affective (meaning "incoming messages) component of pain. Morphine not only decreases the anxiety accompanying pain, but it usually produces a sensation of well-being and euphoria.

(2) Respiration

Morphine acts as a continuous depressant of the automatic respiration center in the brain. In man, death from narcotics is usually caused by respiratory arrest.

(3) Pupils

Morphine causes constriction of the pupils of the eyes. A person who has taken a dose of narcotics will have characteristic "pin point pupils", that is, pupils which are much smaller in size than normal and react poorly to light. This is due to an action on the oculo-motor nerve (the nerve controlling diameter of the pupil). It is important to note that neither meperidine (Demerol®) nor pentazocine (Talwin®) cause significant pupillary constriction so that pin-point pupils are not a distinguishing characteristic of Demerol® or Talwin® users.

(4) Emetic or Vomiting Effects

The initial effect of morphine is to cause nausea and vomiting. When taken orally, the narcotics have a direct effect on the stomach by causing abdominal distress and vomiting. However, even when the narcotics are injected, feelings of nausea and vomiting may occur. This is due to the fact that the narcotics stimulate a center in the brain called the chemo-trigger receptor zone (CTZ). The CTZ is responsible for the nausea and vomiting someone experiences when exposed to noxious chemicals. Alcohol also stimulates this area in the brain. Stimulation of the CTZ occurs relatively early in the course of narcotic effect on the body. Later during the course of a single dose of narcotic, another area in the brain called the vomiting center is suppressed so that it becomes difficult to even induce vomiting.

(5) Excitation

In very high doses, the narcotics can cause convulsions. There are three narcotics which are especially known to cause this problem and they are Demerol®, Darvon®, and Talwin®. Some people also have a paradoxical response to the narcotics and instead of experiencing sed-ation, stimulation results. This occurs in several animal species and well, and in fact, morphine has been used on race horses to make them run faster.

(6) REM Sleep

Sleep time can be increased with morphine use in people who nor-mally can't sleep well due to pain. However as a general rule, morphine causes a decrease in REM sleep and a decrease in total sleep time in general even though it may cause drowsiness.

B. Heart and Blood Vessels

Morphine can cause bradycardia, which is a slowing of heart beat, but this slowing is usually not critical. Morphine also causes a dilation of peripheral blood vessels so that flushing of the skin can result. It is believed that this effect is due to the release of histamine, the body sub-stance which is involved with allergy and which can cause vasodilation (widening of the veins). It is known that at injection sites of morphine, hives may appear due to this histamine release.

The blood vessel dilation may cause hypotension (low blood pressure) and this effect can be markedly increased with the simultaneous use of phenothiazine drugs such as chlorpromazine (Thorazine®) or prochlor-perazine (Compazine®).

C. Gastrointestinal system

Morphine and other narcotics cause a delay in the passage of food through the gastrointestinal system. The intestines may have an increased movement activity but the movement is more of a spasm and the stomach or intestinal contents are not propelled along the tract properly. Since the intestinal contents remain in the bowel for so long, more water than normal is absorbed out of the colon and constipation can result. This constipation can be a very difficult problem, especially in older people, and it can be very difficult to treat. These effects on the bowel caused by narcotics may be due to a local release of serotonin.

D. Kidneys

Morphine causes an increase in the release of anti-diuretic hormone in the body with the result that there is also a decrease in the effectiveness of diuretics ("water pills") especially when given to people with heart trouble.

E. **SUMMARY** (Pharmacology of Narcotic Analgesics)

—The mechanism of action of the narcotic analgesics appears at least in part to involve their binding with receptors in the brain which are involved with the body's feelings and response to pain.

—In general, the narcotic analgesics affect the following organ systems:
- —CNS- causing pain relief, respiratory depression, pupillary constriction, stimulation of nausea and vomiting in lower doses, suppression of nausea and vomiting at very high doses, seizuring in high doses, and a decrease in REM sleep time.
- —Heart and blood vessels- slowing of the heart, and drop in blood pressure.
- —Gastrointestinal system- constipation.
- —Kidneys- minor decrease in urine production.

3. ADVERSE REACTIONS

The most common adverse reactions, or side effects of the narcotic analgesics are:
- —Nausea, vomiting, and dizziness. (These effects can be minimized if a person lays down.)
- —Mental clouding.

—Dysphoria (a feeling of unpleasantness) is experienced by some people, instead of euphoria.

—Constipation

—Pain sensitivity, or an increase in awareness of pain can occur after the medication has worn off.

—Perforation of the nasal septum, or the skin between the nostrils, can be caused by heroin "snorting". Regular cocaine and methamphetamine use can also cause this problem.

—Allergic reactions, manifested as hives can appear at or near injection sites due to a release of histamine in the body.

—Respiratory depression in newborns can occur when the narcotics are given to the mother during labor and delivery. Respiratory depression in adults can also be a problem, especially in people who already have some other respiratory problem such as emphysema, obesity, etc.

4. TOLERANCE

A high degree of tolerance is produced to morphine's analgesia, euphoria, sedation, respiratory depression, hypotension, and nausea and vomiting. Tolerance develops to a moderate degree to the slowed heart beat, but it doesn't develop at all to the pupillary constriction, constipation and convulsive effects. Thus, even a long-term user will still be plagued by constipation and will always have the characteristic pin-point pupils.

Since tolerance develops to the effects of respiratory depression, which is the usual cause of death, the lethal level continues to rise with increased usage. These are the only drugs of abuse where the lethal level continually remains above the level of chronic usage, no matter what dosage level is reached. However, the key words in that statement are "chronic usage" since any period of abstinence appears to decrease tolerance. This means that if a user stops using narcotic for a period of time, their "usual dose" of narcotic before abstinence may suddenly be a lethal dose since their tolerance, and therefore the lethal level, will have decreased.

5. WITHDRAWAL AND PHYSICAL DEPENDENCE

The narcotics cause the development of a physical dependence and with abrupt discontinuance of usage, a narcotic withdrawal syndrome will occur. The severity of the withdrawal will depend on a number of factors which include the type of narcotic used, the amount and duration of use, and the general health of the person.

Withdrawal from morphine or heroin will begin between 8 and 12 hours after the last dose with the onset of tearing, yawning, sweating, and runny nose. At about 12 to 14 hours, the person may fall into a restless sleep which may last several hours. Upon awakening, the person will most likely feel worse than before. As the withdrawal progresses, the pupils become dilated, there is a loss of appetite, and the person is restless, irritable, and tremulous. As the syndrome reaches full intensity at about 48 to 72 hours, there is increasing irritability, insomnia, violent yawning, marked loss of appetite, severe sneezing, tearing, and runny nose. Weakness and depression are common, as are nausea, vomiting, and diarrhea. Excessive sweating plus waves of gooseflesh occur, the latter being the basis of the expression "cold turkey". There are bone and muscle pain, and also involuntary muscle jerks and kicks which gave rise to the term "kicking the habit". Most of these symptoms disappear within 7 to 10 days, but there is a period of a "protracted abstinence syndrome" which may last for weeks. During this time there are certain physiologic abnormalities as well as a high incidence of stress intolerance, low self-image, and an overconcern about discomfort. This is a critical time and relapse occurs commonly during this period.

Methadone withdrawal may not start until 24 to 48 hours after the last dose. The symptoms will peak at about the third day and may not decrease until about the third week. The acute withdrawal from methadone may continue to six or seven weeks and the protracted withdrawal syndrome may last as long as 24 weeks.

Meperidine withdrawal has an onset of as little as three hours after the last dose and reaches intensity at about 8 to 12 hours. The pupils may not be widely dilated and there is usually little nausea, vomiting, or diarrhea. However, at peak intensity, the muscle twitching, irritability, and nervousness may be worse than with morphine withdrawal. Few symptoms are visible after about the fourth of fifth day.

Withdrawal from all narcotics basically follows these same general patterns, however, the shorter acting narcotics usually have a shorter, more intense withdrawal while the narcotics with a longer duration of action produce a more prolonged withdrawal with milder symptoms. Narcotic withdrawal is usually not life-threatening, although a marked electrolyte (potassium, sodium, chloride, etc.) imbalance caused by excessive vomiting and diarrhea must be watched.

FETAL ADDICTION

Babies of narcotic-using mothers can be born with an addiction to narcotics and a withdrawal syndrome of some degree usually occurs in 80% of these newborns. The symptoms of newborn withdrawal typically begin in the first few days of life and include hyperactivity, irritability, tremors, regurgitation, poor feeding, and diarrhea. Convulsions may occur and appear to be more common in methadone withdrawal than with other narcotics. The reason for newborn withdrawal convulsions, when this event is uncommon in adult withdrawal is unknown, but may have to do with the differences in newborn metabolism and decrease in blood brain barrier protection. Newborn withdrawals are usually not serious and only about 20% of the babies need medical assistance during withdrawal. Decreasing doses of paregoric (a camphorated opium solution) or phenobarbital are frequently used to wean the babies.

There appears to be no significant birth deformity causing (teratogenic) effects with the use of narcotics. Any problems are usually caused by poor maternal nutrition and prenatal care. Babies born to addicted mothers have consistently low birth weights, but it still has not been conclusively determined if this is due to poor prenatal care or to an actual effect of the drug itself.

No studies have, as yet, been undertaken to evaluate the long-term effects of fetal addiction, but research in this area is definitely needed to determine the extent of physiological and psychological damage which might result from the passive addiction of the fetus to a narcotic drug and the traumatic withdrawal which is experienced so soon in life.

6. COMPLICATIONS OF INTRAVENOUS DRUG ABUSE

HEPATITIS

Viral hepatitis can be easily transmitted by the sharing of intravenous injection sets with an infected person. Hepatitis is the most common cause of hospitalization of heroin abusers.

ADULTERANTS

Adulterants, (or excipient ingredients) are usually pharmacologically inactive ingredients added to a drug to give it bulk (some drugs are active in quantities as small as a few grains of salt), or as preservatives, or as a "glue" to hold other ingredients together in a tablet. Other excipient ingredients include coloring agents, sugar or wax coatings, or flavorings. Excipients such as quinine, procaine and lidocaine are often used to cut heroin. Quinine has been implicated in low platelet count (thrombocytopenia) and severe bleeding disorders seen in addicts.

Until recently, some heroin abusers used a combination of Pyribenzamine® (tripelennamine) and Talwin® (pentazocine) as replacement for heroin when supplies were short. Pyribenzamine® comes in tablet form and is crushed and combined with crushed Talwin® tablets and injected. The Pyribenzamine® tablets contain blue-dye talc and when this insoluble substance is injected into a vein, it eventually becomes lodged in the small blood vessels of the lungs. This can cause problems in the lungs and also in the heart as it tries to pump blood through all the clogged blood vessels of the lungs. This problem is called "blue velvet lung" because at autopsy the lung will appear to have a blue, velvety appearance. In recent years, the use of Talwin® and Pyribenzamine® (often referred to as T's and blues, for Talwin® and the blue tripelennamine) became so wide spread as a substitute for heroin, that the manufacturer of Talwin® sought to limit the ability to abuse Talwin® tablets. In 1983, Talwin® tablets were replaced by a product called Talwin-NX®. The NX portion stands for naloxone, which is a narcotic antagonist. (Naloxone will be discussed later in the chapter.) Naloxone, is inactivated in stomach acid, and is only active if given intravenously (I.V.). Heroin addicts, using Talwin® as a temporary substitute in hard times dissolve the Talwin®, and inject it intravenously. (An injectable Talwin® is also available, but it is much more difficult to obtain.) When Talwin-NX® tabs are injected intravenously, the naloxone works as an antagonist, and very little effect can be felt. Also, it may precipitate withdrawal. However when Talwin-NX® is taken orally, the naloxone is inactivated, and only Talwin® is available for absorption.

7. LEVO ALPHA ACETYLMETHADOL (LAAM)

Methadone has a duration of action of about 25 hours. Patients on methadone maintenance are either required to go into a clinic daily to receive a dose or a 3 to 4 day supply is given to the person per visit. This latter method can lead to a number of problems such as overdoses in the patient, children, etc., or selling the methadone on the street.

LAAM is a long-acting type of methadone which may be able to solve some of these problems. LAAM can suppress narcotic withdrawal symptoms for approximately 72 hours. It is metabolized in the liver to pharmacologically active metabolites which are at least in part responsible for its prolonged duration of action. An 80mg dose of LAAM given three times a week is approximately equal to 100mg/day of methadone. When LAAM is given to people who are not opiate tolerant, it produces typical narcotic effects, including analgesia and lethargy, but it has a much slower onset of action than methadone. The slower onset prevents the feeling of a drug "rush" from occurring and this makes LAAM less attractive for abuse.

As with methadone, overdose with LAAM is potentially lethal, but with the type of program of giving only one dose every three days or so, there will be less of a problem with drug stockpiling as can occur with methadone programs. However, if overdose does occur, it may be more difficult to manage due to the very long duration of action of LAAM.

SUMMARY (Tolerance, Withdrawal, Complications)

—Tolerance develops to pain relief, euphoria, sleep, breathing depression, hypotension, and nausea, but not to pupillary constriction, constipation, and seizure effects.

—Withdrawal is usally marked by pupillary dilation, irritablility, insomnia, decreased appetite, runny nose, diarrhea, nausea, and sweating. Fetal addiction and withdrawal may occur from maternal use during pregnancy.

—The possible complications of IV narcotic abuse include hepatitis and adverse effects on the blood.

Although heroin is the most notorious drug of this group there is increasing use of other pain relief medicines. Patients must be carfully evaluated and monitored in order to provide care. It is beyond the intent of this almanac to discuss the treatment issues involved in getting patients off pain medicine.

There is still controversy over the use of methadone and other drugs such as LAAM which are used in helping to get patients off heroin. Needless to say, each patient should be carefully monitored and there should be active physician involvement no matter which drugs have been used.

CHAPTER THREE-B:

NARCOTIC ANTAGONISTS

There are certain receptor sites in the body with which the narcotics can bind (sometimes called enkephalin receptor sites) and with this binding they cause the typical narcotic action. Other drugs, however, have been found which can bind with the narcotic receptors and they cause no action at all. In fact, when these drugs are present in the body, not only will they block the binding of the narcotics to the receptor sites, but they prevent or stop the actions of the narcotics. These drugs are called "narcotic antagonists" since they prevent or stop the actions of the narcotics. The narcotic antagonists were first developed and used to reverse the effects of a narcotic overdose. A person who is in a coma or severe respiratory depression due to an excessive narcotic dose can be brought back to consciousness immediately by the administration of a narcotic antagonist. Of course, a narcotic antagonist will not be able to reverse any brain damage which might have already occurred due to respiratory arrest and lack of oxygen to the brain. The narcotic antagonists have also proved their worth in the case of babies born with respiratory depression due to a dose of narcotic administered to the mother for pain during labor. An interesting usage of the narcotic antagonists, which has for the most part been stopped now, was as a diagnostic tool for narcotic addiction. When a narcotic antagonist is administered to a narcotic dependent person, a withdrawal syndrome can be induced, thus confirming the dependency. Smaller doses can also be administered which would reverse any "pin point pupils" present and thus also confirm narcotic usage. However, since a withdrawal induced by a narcotic antagonist is usually extremely abrupt and intense in onset, this practice has been questioned ethically and generally discontinued.

One of the first narcotic antagonists which was widely used was nalorphine, which was sold under the trade name of Nalline®. Nalline® has been proven to be highly effective in reversing the respiratory depression of narcotic overdose. Nalline®, however, is not an ideal narcotic antagonist since it can also exhibit narcotic-like respiratory depression in high doses. Narcotic usage also had to be almost definitely proven before Nalline® was administered to comatose patients, because if it was accidently given to someone who had actually overdosed on a sedative-hypnotic drug, the respiratory depression would be severely increased instead of reversed. Nalline® is said to be a narcotic agonist-antagonist since it has both the properties of narcotic action (agonistic) and properties which stop narcotic action (antagonistic). It is now recognized that almost all narcotics have some degree of antagonistic properties although their agonistic properties are usually dominant. It was also found that Nalline® is not very effective in treating overdoses caused by those narcotics which have a high antagonistic capability of their own, such as pentazocine (Talwin®). When Talwin®, or a similar drug is given in large doses to someone who is morphine or heroin dependent, a narcotic withdrawal syndrome can be induced.

The real breakthrough in narcotic antagonist therapy came with the discovery of naloxone or Narcan®. Narcan® was the first "pure" narcotic antagonist developed and its usage has been highly successful. It has no respiratory depressant action of its own so can be used in large amounts and also without fear in overdose situations of undetermined cause since it cannot worsen even sedative-hypnotic overdoses. Narcan® is also useful in treating overdoses of the agonist-antagonist narcotics such as Talwin®. The only drawback of Narcan® usage is that it is relatively short acting (1 to 3 hours) and care must be taken in narcotic overdose situations to avoid allowing the overdose patient to slip back into coma as the Narcan® wears off. This is especially important with the long-acting narcotics such as methadone which has a duration of approximately 24 hours. Thus, it must be remembered that the narcotic is still within the body, but its actions are temporarily prevented while the antagonist blocks any narcotic binding and therefore activity with the receptor sites.

A new, longer-acting pure narcotic antagonist called naltrexone is currently being used experimentally in this country and will hopefully at least partially overcome the problem of the shorter acting Narcan®. Naltrexone has another advantage over Narcan®, in that it is effective orally. Narcan® is well absorbed from the stomach, however, after that it passes immediately through the liver, where it is made inactive by adding glucuronide. This immediate inactivation does not occur as extensively with naltrexone, so it is active in oral form. Several studies indicate that 50 or 60mg of naltrexone given orally can block the effects of narcotic analgesics in humans for a full day (24 hours). This therapy may prove useful for treatment of narcotic dependent persons who have already withdrawn from narcotics. Naltrexone would be contraindicated in acute withdrawal, because it could precipitate sudden and severe narcotic withdrawal symptoms. In clinical studies, heroin dependent persons who had undergone treatment and were maintained on naltrexone were unable to get desired euphoric effects when they tried to return to heroin.

Another recent trend in the treatment of narcotic dependent persons is the use of clonidine during the acute withdrawal phase. Clonidine is a medication commonly used to treat hypertension (high blood pressure). While its use is controversial, some treatment centers have reported success with the use of clonidine in treating the physical symptoms of narcotic analgesic withdrawal. Clonidine does not produce euphoric effects, and does not act at an enkephalin receptor site. It acts on a type of receptor called a central alpha-noradrenergic receptor. When clonidine is taken, blood pressure drops, heart rate slows, drowsiness may occur, and with chronic use constipation may occur. These are some of the physical effects seen with withdrawal. One theorized mechanism of action of clonidine in opiate withdrawal is that stimulation of the central alpha-noradrenergic receptor causes it to stimulate release of enkephalins, which in turn stimulate the enkephalin receptor, causing the physical effects mentioned above.

SUMMARY (Narcotic antagonists and clonidine):

—Nalorphine was one of the early narcotic antagonists and is rarely used now because it exhibits respiratory depression in high doses.

—Naloxone was the first pure narcotic antagonist. It is currently considered to be the treatment of choice for narcotic overdose.

—Naltrexone is longer acting than Narcan®, and is being used in oral form in narcotic treatment centers.

—Clonidine is not a narcotic antagonist, but has been found by some to be a useful adjunct in the treatment of narcotic analgesic abstinence.

The narcotic antagonists are drugs which specifically block the effects of narcotic analgesics, and are used to help awaken patients who have overdosed.

CHAPTER 4

Psychomotor Stimulants

PSYCHOMOTOR STIMULANTS

INTRODUCTION

HISTORY

The psychomotor stimulants include the amphetamines, cocaine, and methylphenidate (Ritalin®). The effects of amphetamine were first investigated in 1927, in an attempt to find a drug useful in the treatment of asthma. It was found to be helpful in the treatment of asthma, however with many side effects. Following World War II, its abuse as a psychomotor stimulant became more and more frequent.

Cocaine comes from the leaves of a plant called Erythroxylon coca, native to Peru and Bolivia. The leaves have been chewed since before the Spanish colonized Latin America, by the Inca Indians. In the late nineteenth century, and first decade of the twentieth century, cocaine became a popular ingredient of many patent medicines and tonics, including Coca-Cola. (Don't worry, it has not been in Coca-Cola since 1903.) Cocaine became a useful agent for surgical anesthesia, particularly of the nose, throat, and eye, around the beginning of the twentieth century.

. Methylphenidate (Ritalin®) was first synthesized in 1944 and is chemically related to the amphetamines. Its major medical use is in the treatment of hyperactive children (this will be discussed later), however, just as others in this class, it is frequently abused for its stimulant properties.

CHEMISTRY

Cocaine is not chemically related to the amphetamines or Ritalin®, however, many effects are similar.

DRUG	T 1/2 (hours)	DURATION
amphetamines	5-20	*see below
methylphenidate (Ritalin®)	2-7	6 hours
cocaine	1-5	short

*Amphetamines have large variations in half-life and duration, because their excretion is largely dependent on urine pH (acidity).

EPIDEMIOLOGY

Amphetamine use has declined in recent years since a peak of use around 1972. A recent, and dangerous twist to amphetamine abuse is the emergence of amphetamine "look alikes" which can be sold in any retail outlet legally in most states. These will be discussed in greater detail later in the chapter.

Illicit cocaine use tripled in the period between 1972 and 1980. By 1980, 32 million Americans in the 18-to 25 year old age group (or around 27.5%) had tried cocaine. Another study indicated that 16% of the high school graduating class of 1981 had tried cocaine. Cocaine currently sells for between $75 and $160 per gram on the street, and this is for samples which usually range in purity from 15-60%. Usually, at least a 25-100mg dose (there are 1000mg in one gram) of pure cocaine is required for euphoric effect.

CLINICAL USES

—Amphetamines and Ritalin®:
* *—control of appetite, weight reduction
* —control of narcolepsy (sudden attacks of sleep)
* —control of hyperkinetic behavior in children
* —antagonize effects of depressants
* *—treat mild depression
* *—relief of, or prevention of fatigue

—Cocaine:
* —local anesthetic for surgical procedures on eye, nose, throat, ear, rectum, vagina
* **—ingredient in pain coctails in terminal cancer victims

*amphetamines and Ritalin® are considered poor choices for treating these disorders
**the usefulness of cocaine in pain cocktails is questionable

This chapter will first discuss the amphetamines and Ritalin®, and then will discuss cocaine separately.

AMPHETAMINES AND METHYLPHENIDATE

1. BIOPHARMACEUTICS

ABSORPTION

The amphetamines are ionized in the acidity of the stomach. This means that they have decreased lipid solubility under these conditions so that little absorption occurs in the stomach. Note in the illustration below that the amphetamines become un-ionized in the alkaline intestines and can be rapidly absorbed at that point. Peak blood levels will occur in approximately one hour if there is no food in the stomach to delay the drug from reaching the intestine.

Methylphenidate (Ritalin®) is also fairly well absorbed when taken orally since it is also lipid soluble.

ABSORPTION OF AMPHETAMINES

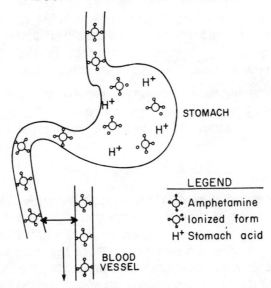

STOMACH

LEGEND
- Amphetamine
- Ionized form
H^+ Stomach acid

BLOOD VESSEL

DISTRIBUTION

The amphetamines are quite lipid soluble, and, after absorption they distribute into organs such as the brain, lung, and kidney. The amphetamines cross the blood brain barrier very readily. Central nervous system effects are seen within 30 minutes of an oral dose and the action will last for several hours. Brain levels reach about 10 times the blood levels and this high concentration in the brain accounts for the relatively great CNS effect. Little is known of the distribution pattern of Ritalin®, except that it gains easy access to the brain since central nervous system activity is definitely seen.

METABOLISM

In an acidic urine, around 70% of an amphetamine dose is excreted without being metabolized. Another substantial amount is conjugated with a water soluble glucuronide molecule and inactivated. Some of the metabolites of the amphetamines, however, are still active. About 6-10% of methamphetamine is metabolized to amphetamine. Amphetamine itself is principally metabolized to para-hydroxyamphetamine which has much less of a central nervous system effect than amphetamine, but it can cause an increase in blood pressure. Amphetamine is also metabolized to a small extent to a methoxy (CH_3O-) derivative which has hallucinogenic activity. When the urine is less acidic and more alkaline, a larger percentage of amphetamine is metabolized, and will be eliminated more slowly. A greater incidence of toxic effects can be seen under these conditions. (These chemical reactions are illustrated in the appendix).

Ritalin® is partially excreted unchanged, but the major metabolite is ritalinic acid. Ritalinic acid is very poorly lipid soluble so it cannot cross the blood brain barrier and therefore has little central nervous system effect.

EXCRETION

The major method of excretion is through the urine. A large amount of the amphetamines are excreted unchanged. The exact amount that is excreted unchanged is dependent on the acidity of the urine. At the normal acidity of the urine, as much as 60% of the drug will be excreted unchanged within 48 hours, since the amphetamines are much more water soluble under acidic conditions. As mentioned in the "metabolism" section, if the urine is made slightly alkaline, as can occur with certain foods or by excessive sodium bicarbonate intake, only 2 to 3% of the drug will be excreted unchanged in the urine within 48 hours. If the drug remains unexcreted for so long, greater metabolism can occur. Since some of the metabolites have undersirable effects (such as the methoxy metabolite which causes hallucinations) the increased metabolism could cause an increase in drug complications. In fact, the hallucinations and drug-induced psychoses which can occur with amphetamine use, were shown to be much worse and more prolonged when the urine was made alkaline by ingestion of large amounts of baking soda or soda crackers.

Ritalin® is mostly excreted in the urine also.

SUMMARY (Biopharmaceutics of amphetamines):

The amphetamines and methylphenidate are well absorbed from the alkaline environment of the intestines. They are rapidly distributed across the brain barrier and have very potent effects on the brain. Some of the metabolites of the amphetamines are active and can cause high blood pressure and hallucinations if present in sufficient quantity. Metabolism and excretion are both affected by acidity of the urine. When the urine is more acid, amphetamines are excreted more rapidly. When it is more alkaline, more metabolites are formed, and excretion occurs relatively slowly.

2. PHARMACOLOGY

MECHANISM OF ACTION

At this point, a review of the sections discussing nerves and neurotransmitters, and the autonomic nervous system in the introductory chapter is advised.

The actions of the psychomotor stimulants are basically confined to the central and peripheral nervous systems. They act through the release and/or increase in the effects of neurotransmitters.

In the central nervous system, the psychomotor stimulants act through the neurotransmitters dopamine and norepinephrine. It appears that an increase in dopamine in parts of the brain where dopamine is excitatory is responsible for much of the central nervous system effect that is seen. There are several mechanisms by which these drugs achieve this increase in dopamine. The amphetamines seem to cause the release of newly synthesized dopamine from the pre-synaptic nerve to stimulate the receptors on the post synaptic nerve. Ritalin® also releases dopamine from pre-synaptic nerves, but it seems to release dopamine from stored pools rather than newly synthesized dopamine. Also contributing to the action of the amphetamines is inhibition of the action of MAO, the enzyme which ends the action of norepinephrine and dopamine in the synapse, and inhibition of re-uptake of these transmitters back into pre-synaptic nerves. This allows norepinephrine and dopamine to remain active in the synapse longer.

MECHANISM OF ACTION OF AMPHETAMINES AND METHYLPHENIDATE

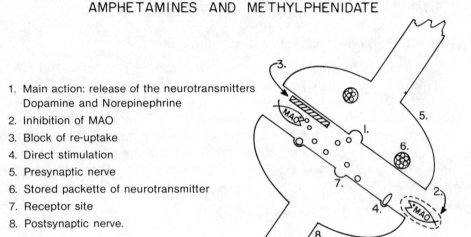

1. Main action: release of the neurotransmitters Dopamine and Norepinephrine
2. Inhibition of MAO
3. Block of re-uptake
4. Direct stimulation
5. Presynaptic nerve
6. Stored packette of neurotransmitter
7. Receptor site
8. Postsynaptic nerve.

𝟬–Amphetamine

o–Transmitter

    In the peripheral nervous system, norepinephrine is the neuro-transmitter involved in the stimulant action. Norepinephrine is a neuro-transmitter which acts in the sympathetic nervous system (SNS). With the stimulation by norepinephrine, the SNS becomes the dominant portion of the autonomic nervous system. Thus, the typical "fight or flight" response is elicited with psychomotor stimulant use. Since the psychomotor stimulants do cause the sympathetic nervous system to dominate, they are called sympathomimetic drugs (ie. their action "mimics" the action of the SNS). The amphetamines and Ritalin® both seem to act by similar mechanisms in the peripheral nervous system. They seem to directly cause the release of norepinephrine from the pre-synaptic nerve endings. They also inhibit the re-uptake of norepinephrine back into the pre-synaptic nerves, and to block MAO, thus increasing the effect of norepinephrine. Some of the stimulants may also be able to directly stim-ulate the peripheral post-synaptic nerve receptors themselves.

ORGAN SYSTEM EFFECTS

1. Central nervous system:
   —Euphoria, confidence, elation
   —Relief from fatigue, increased mental alertness
   —Suppression of appetite through depression of the feeding center
   —Increased motor and speech activity
   —Increased temperature due to an action on the temperature regulation center in the brain

2. Peripheral nervous system (due to stimulation of the SNS by increased norepinephrine activity):
   —Increased respiration rate
   —Increased blood pressure and heart rate at high doses, however, sometimes at lower doses, the heart rate is decreased, because of a reflex action which causes the heart rate to slow when blood pressure is increased
   —Decreased gastrointestinal activity which can cause constipation
   —Urinary retention

3. A very curious effect of the amphetamines, and particularly of Ritalin®, is the paradoxical effect on hyperkinetic behavior disorder in children (also called minimal brain dysfunction, or MBD). MBD is marked by short attention span, purposeless hyperactivity, impulsiveness, overreaction in emotional situations, learning deficits, and perceptual deficits. The exact mechanism of MBD is not known, however, it is believed that it is caused by either an abnormal metabolism or an imbalance of certain neurotransmitters in specific parts of the brain. The neurotransmitters involved are acetylcholine, norepinephrine, serotonin, and dopamine. It is believed that Ritalin®, and the amphetamines, by increasing brain levels of dopamine have the paradoxical effect quieting hyperkinetic children. In fact, Ritalin® has proven effective in 75% of MBD children for controlling hyperactivity and impulsive behavior resulting in learning impairments.

SUMMARY (Pharmacology of amphetamines):

The amphetamines and methylphenidate are sympathetic nervous system and central nervous system stimulants. Among their effects are, increased motor activity, increased alertness, decreased appetite, increased body temperature, increased respiration and heart rate, increased blood pressure, constipation, and urinary retention.

3. TOLERANCE

Tolerance does develop to certain of the actions of the psychomotor stimulants such as the euphoria, appetite suppression, and heart and blood pressure effects. Tolerance also occurs to a certain extent to wakefulness and hyperactivity. Cross-tolerance between cocaine and the other psychomotor stimulants has not been shown to exist, although there is cross-tolerance between the amphetamine-like drugs (ie. a person tolerant to amphetamine would most likely be tolerant to Ritalin®, but not to cocaine).

4. WITHDRAWAL

It has long been argued whether physiological or only psychological dependence developed with prolonged stimulant use. It is now clearly known that a period of depression, fatigue, increased appetite, and prolonged sleep, accompanied by REM rebound follows the cessation of stimulant use. This is usually only apparent in people on large doses of psychomotor stimulants for a long time. This withdrawal seems to parallel a time of dopamine and norepinephrine depletion as demonstrated by a drop in the excretion of their metabolites. The withdrawal from the psychomotor stimulants is not as dramatic or life-threatening as sedative-hypnotic or even narcotic withdrawal, but the withdrawal state does exist.

5. ACUTE TOXICITY AND DEATH

With large doses of the psychomotor stimulants, extreme sympathomimetic effects occur. These effects would include very rapid heart beat, hypertension, headache, profuse sweating, and severe chest pain. With severe intoxication, delirium, panic, paranoia, and hallucination can also be present. With amphetamine-like drugs death can occur due to extreme heat elevation, convulsions, and finally circulatory collapse.

6. COMPLICATIONS FROM THE ROUTES OF ADMINISTRATION

All of the psychomotor stimulants can be used intravenously (IV). Therefore, all of the complications of IV use can occur, such as transfer of hepatitis and other communicable diseases, as well as ulceration and infection of injection sites. Because amphetamines are often mixed with basic substances (ie. sodium bicarbonate) to increase absorption, one can get alkali burns with IV use. The stimulants are often also "snorted" (especially cocaine) and habitual usage in this manner can result in perforation and ulceration of the nasal septum.

7. **CHRONIC USE**

With chronic use of amphetamines exceeding 50-100mg per day, an interesting phenomenon of "amphetamine psychosis" frequently occurs. These persons start out usually with paranoid ideations, which, initially they can intellectually realize as being delusional. The person may also start exhibiting stereotypic behavior which is purposeless, but repeated endlessly. One example is a girl who polished and removed the polish from her nails repeatedly until they were raw and bleeding. Eventually the person will no longer be able to differentiate between reality and delusion and a full blown psychosis develops which is clinically indistinguishable from paranoid schizophrenia. There will be many paranoid delusions, aggressive behavior and hallucinations which are usually visual, but may be auditory or tactile. The psychosis will generally clear when amphetamine use is ceased, however, if the implication of drug use is missed, problems can result. There have been case reports of amphetamine users being given shock treatment and numerous antipsychotic medications which mysteriously did not improve the condition until it was discovered that the patient was actually in a state of amphetamine induced psychosis, and were continuing their drug intake. Amphetamine psychosis can be induced in people without prior major psychopathology and the amphetamines have been shown to worsen existing psychotic tendency, resulting in permanent psychosis.

8. **"LOOK-A-LIKES" AND ADULTERANTS**

The problem of substitution of inexpensive, easily obtainable, drugs for those which are more costly, illegal, or otherwise more difficult to obtain exists in all classes of drugs of abuse. However nowhere is it more true, than with the psychomotor stimulants (including cocaine). Illegally manufactured amphetamine usually contains 2mg or less (if any) amphetamine. Most often, the additional active ingredients in amphetamine samples are caffeine, strychnine, various decongestant medications, or acetaminophen (Tylenol®). Most of the pharmaceutical manufacturer (licit) amphetamine tablets range in potency from 5mg to 15mg. The danger in taking tablets which are "look-a-likes" to real amphetamines, or illicit amphetamines containing adulterants, is that overdose may accidentally result when real amphetamine is taken. For example, a user may normally take 12 "crosstops" (a term for a type of illicit amphetamine) each tablet containing only 1mg of amphetamine along with some caffeine and ephedrine. However, if he unknowingly obtains tablets of a more potent variety, containing 5mg of amphetamine, he could easily overdose, if he takes the former number of tablets.

SUMMARY (Tolerance, withdrawal, toxicity):

Most psychomotor stimulants are short acting, have a brief effect and there is a much greater need to increase the dose than with other psychoactive drugs. These drugs are the only "uppers" that people become dependent on. Withdrawal is short in duration and not intense but is often complicated with withdrawal from alcohol and other "downers".

CHAPTER FOUR-B:

COCAINE

1. BIOPHARMACEUTICS

Cocaine is well absorbed from all mucous membranes. Orally administered cocaine is mostly hydrolyzed (a type of metabolism) in the stomach
to an inactive product called ecgonine (see appendix for chemical structures). Most of the cocaine that is absorbed from the gastrointestinal tract
is immediately metabolized on first pass through the liver. However, small
amounts of activity can still be seen if doses of around 150mg or greater
are taken orally. The major route of administration of cocaine, at least in
the U.S., is insufflation ("snorting") which results in absorption through
nasal membranes. Since the drug immediately enters the blood circulation without first going through the liver, a sufficient blood level of active
drug can be reached to obtain a drug effect.

Another common route of administration is through absorption in the
buccal or cheek cavity. Drugs can also be directly absorbed into the main
circulation from this membrane area and again bypass liver metabolism.
This is the method used by the many South American Indians who still
chew coca leaves like their ancestors, the Incas. In the traditional
method, the Indians also chew lime with the cocaine to create an alkaline
environment in their mouths. This increases absorption and thus
increases the onset of action.

Absorption of cocaine from any mucous membranes, such as the
inside of the nose, or cheek, is controlled by the degree of blood vessel
constriction which occurs, caused by the cocaine. Since absorption in
these areas occurs directly across a membrane into a small blood
vessel surface.

Cocaine gains easy and rapid access to the CNS, and effects from
"snorted" cocaine can be seen within 15 minutes. High concentrations
are also seen in the spleen, kidney, and pancreas.

Cocaine is rapidly metabolized by <u>hydrolysis</u> (this process "chops" off
a portion of the molecule) in the liver and in the serum to benzoylecgonine and ecgonine, both which are inactive. Cocaine is mostly
excreted as benzoylecgonine and ecgonine in the urine. Less than 20%
of cocaine is excreted unchanged.

2. PHARMACOLOGY

Cocaine affects the autonomic nervous system in a manner similar to the amphetamines. It exerts it action by decreasing reuptake of norepinephrine at the synapse, thereby increasing its effects. Cocaine works by similar action in the central nervous system, except that there it blocks reuptake of dopamine. Cocaine has an additional action, not seen in the other psychomotor stimulants. It exerts a local anesthetic action on nerve-cell membranes, and prevents generation and conduction of nerve impulses. When applied to mucous membranes or injected into nerves, a transient numbness results. Because of cocaine's ability to cause blood vessel constriction, it was quite popular as an agent for surgeries, nasal surgery especially, since not only does it have the anesthetic action, but surgical bleeding is minimized. Cocaine is still used to a certain extent in this context, but its high abuse potential has caused many doctors to use other methods rather than keep cocaine supplies around.

3. **TOLERANCE.** There is some controversy concerning the development of tolerance to cocaine since many researchers feel that tolerance to cocaine does not occur. However, tolerance may occur to a certain extent since extremely large doeses (i.e. 10gm) can be tolerated in chronic users, whereas these amounts could be lethal to a naive individual.

4. **WITHDRAWAL.** Symptoms are similar to those of the amphetamines and Ritalin®. Withdrawal from cocaine sometimes leaves a person in a deeply depressed state called "Cocaine Blues".

5. **TOXICITY AND DEATH.** Toxic signs are similar to those of amphetamines. Death from cocaine may occur due to respiratory depression since high doses of cocaine essentially anesthetize or "numb" the respiratory center in the brain.

6. **COMPLICATIONS FROM ROUTES OF ADMINISTRATION.** Cocaine, like the amphetamines can cause ulceration and perforation of the nasal septum when habitually "snorted". This is because the tiny blood vessels in the tissue which cocaine contacts are constricted, and that tissue loses it blood supply.

A recent and hazardous trend is smoking of "freebase" cocaine. "Freebase" cocaine is made from the ordinary form, cocaine hydrochloride, by a process involving heating flammable solvents such as ether. The resulting product, cocaine "freebase", can be smoked in a water pipe, or sprinkled on marijuana or tobacco cigarettes. Cocaine "freebase" is effective when smoked, whereas the hydrochloride salt (the usual form) is not. A more intense euphoric effect is felt from smoking "freebase" (as compared with "snorting"). As well as more intense euphoric effects, more intense toxic effects are seen with "freebase", and these include the peripheral as well as CNS effects.

7. **CHRONIC USE.** Cocaine psychosis can occur with chronic use, and appears to be similar to amphetamine psychosis.

SUMMARY (Cocaine):

There seems to be increasing awareness of cocaine use within the last five years. Most persons still "snort" cocaine, although use of free base is becoming more popular because it provides a more intense effect (although with more severe side effects). The effects of cocaine are very similar to those of amphetamine, with the exception that cocaine has the additional action of being a local anesthetic. The use of cocaine is expensive and is seen more in above average income families.

CHAPTER 5

Perceptual Distorters
(Psychedelics)

CHAPTER FIVE:

PERCEPTUAL DISTORTERS (Psychedelics)

These drugs are difficult to categorize, because wide chemical differences exist, because they have greatly differing physical effects, and because even the perceptual effects differ from one drug to another. In many ways, this is a "catch-all" category, and even its title is controversial. In addition to being called "perceptual distorters", many give them the title "hallucinogens", some "psychotomimetic drugs", and others "psychedelic drugs".

The use of perceptual distorters (LSD in particular) increased in the 1960's, with a peak in popularity around 1972. Use then declined until 1977, when there was a renewed increase in popularity.

The use of PCP has greatly increased in recent years, probably because of its relatively low cost and easy ability to manufacture. A 1978 study found that 1 in 8 persons in the 18-to-25 year old group, and 1 in 20 persons in the 12-to-17 year old group had used at least once. In all, 7 million Americans have tried PCP. Another finding was that 23% of those exposed went on to become chronic users. Many injuries are attributable to PCP. Also, in a study of drugs associated with emergency room visits and deaths from January through December of 1979, PCP and PCP in combination with other drugs ranked 5th.

LSD will be considered the prototype for this discussion (covered in chapter 5A). The other major hallucinogens will be briefly discussed in chapter 5B, with the exception of PCP, which will be discussed in chapter 5C.

CHAPTER FIVE-A:

LYSERGIC ACID DIETHYLAMIDE (LSD)

1. INTRODUCTION

LSD is a semisynthetic derivative of the ergot alkaloids obtained from Claviceps purpurea, the fungus that grows on various types of grains, especially rye and also wheat. It is also known as LSD-25 since it was the 25th in a series of compounds studied, and is one of the most potent of all drugs. LSD is active in extremely small amounts. The usual dose ranges from 50 to 300 micrograms which is equivalent to 0.05 to 0.300 milligram, or 0.00005 to 0.0003 gram. When comparing this amount with the weight of an ordinary paper clip, which weighs about 1 gram, it is easy to appreciate the potency of LSD since it is active in such minute quantities. (This would mean that the weight of one paper clip would be equal to the weight of anywhere from 3,333 to 20,000 doses of LSD!)

2. BIOPHARMACEUTICS

Little research has been done on the biopharmaceutics of lysergic acid diethylamide in humans, but it appears to be rapidly and completely absorbed from the GI tract since initial effects are seen within 30 to 40 minutes. LSD readily crosses the blood brain barrier and psychic effects are seen soon after initiation of the drug effect.

LSD is almost completely metabolized in the liver to an inactive oxygenated derivative. The half-life for humans is approximately 1 1/2 hours, however, enough is retained in the CNS to continue psychic effects for 8 to 12 hours.

The major route of excretion appears to be via the bile to the feces so measurement for urinary content would not be accurate. The exact lethal dose for humans has never been determined and no deaths due to LSD toxicity have been reported. It does seem, however, that the lethal dose is inversely proportional to brain size. The LD_{50} (a number representing the dose which is lethal to 50% of the test population) has been determined for several animal species: 46mg of LSD/kg of body weight for mice; 16.5mg/kg for rats; 0.3mg/kg for rabbits, and 0.1mg/kg for one unfortunate elephant. On this basis, the LD_{50} for humans has been calculated to be 0.2mg/kg, or 14mg for a 70kg (154 pound) man.

ABSORPTION/DISTRIBUTION/
METABOLISM/EXCRETION OF LSD

3. PHARMACOLOGY

Much research has been done to determine the mechanism of LSD action but few, if any, definite conclusions have been made. Part of the problem has to do with the research models themselves. Most of the work, out of necessity, has been done with animals and LSD causes a great deal of interspecies differences. It is therefore extremely difficult, if not impossible, to draw correlations to human responses. The other major problem in the study of LSD is that it is intimately linked with the study of brain chemistry and this area of anatomical research is still in its infancy. It is known that LSD definitely affects serotonin areas in the brain by competing with serotonin for post-synaptic receptor sites. It is not known, however, how this effect is modulated by other brain neurotransmitters and which areas of the brain are effected. It is also known that LSD affects some sertonin areas of the brain more than others.

Even though the mechanism(s) of action of LSD is (are) still not understood, the actions themselves have been well documented. The first effects experienced with LSD are usually absent after about six hours. LSD produces effects on both the sympathetic and parasympathetic nervous system, probably from some CNS effect on the autonomic nervous system. Although PSNS symptoms such as salivation, tearing, and occasionally vomiting may occur SNS effects are usually dominant. These effects include dilation of the pupils, increased body temperature, sweating, and appearance of gooseflesh. Blood pressure and heart rate can increase, although these effects are variable. Other miscellaneous physical effects which can occur include tremor, muscle incoordination, and numbness or tingling in the extremities.

The most important of the effects of LSD is of course, the psychic effects. Approximately an hour after ingestion, perceptual alterations gradually appear which eventually become prominent. Somehow there is interference in the influx of the sensory information which results in a distortion of sensory perception. All of the senses are involved but vision seems to be the most affected. Color and texture of items become more vivid and perception of detail, which is normally not noticed, is increased. Afterimages are greatly prolonged and sometimes there is a failure to suppress prior images so that visual overlapping of objects can occur. Many people elaborate on detail of after images to the point of hallucination, but these are usually referred to as "pseudohallucinations" since the user is able to differentiate these images as not being real. True hallucinations, in which the user truely believes in imaginary projections are infrequent at ordinary doses. Auditory hallucinations are even more rare. Sensory input can become so disorganized under the influence of LSD that there can be an overlapping of the various senses. This is known as synesthesia and the user can experience such sensations as "seeing" music or "hearing" color. Other prominent effects seen with LSD are feelings of depersonalization, a loss of body image, and a loss of a sense of reality. The perception of time is distorted and the sense of past, present, and future may be jumbled. Concentration can be difficult and attention can fluctuate rapidly. There is a perfusion of vague ideas and there is often an extreme preoccupation with philosophical issues. This engrossment, coupled with impairments in judgement and illogical thought processes produced by LSD, may cause the user to believe that he has discovered new truths into philosophy or great insights into himself. The descriptions of these "discoveries", however, usually seem unintelligible or nonsensical to those not under LSD influence. Even though many people claim that LSD liberates great artistic insight in writing and painting, these claims too have yet to be proven.

Emotional changes occur with LSD use, but are unpredictable. A mood can shift quickly from intense euphoria to despair, due perhaps only to the fact that the sun went behind a cloud. Also, at times, laughter or tears may occur which are inappropriate to the situation.

Some psychological dependency can occur with LSD use, but no evidence has been found to indicate the development of physical dependency. Tolerance to the physiologic and psychic effects of LSD can and do occur. This tolerance occurs rapidly with use, and disappears rapidly after discontinuation. Cross tolerance between LSD, mescaline, and psilocybin also occurs, indicating possibly a similar mechanism of action for these drugs.

Acute panic reactions can occur with LSD which result in a "bad trip" (or "bummer"). These panic reactions usually occur due to a feeling of imminent danger. If these panic reactions become intense and prolonged, a state of drug-induced psychosis can result. The psychotic episode may be brief or it may last for several years. The mechanism of the LSD action is not known. It may be an unmasking of a previous psychosis, although it is difficult, if not impossible to predict when and with whom such reactions occur.

There is an increased risk of self-destructive behavior with LSD and the other perceptual distorters during either an acute, or a chronic reaction.

"Flashbacks" or spontaneous reoccurrences of an LSD experience can occur without warning for up to a year or longer after LSD use. The exact mechanism of this effect is not known. Since they occur at times when no LSD is in the body, it has been speculated that they represent a behavior that is learned under the influence of LSD-caused psychophysiologic arousal that later can be precipitated under conditions of nervous system arousal. These later conditions could be due to fear, or even the use of stimulants or other drugs such as marijuana.

Much controversy has gone on concerning the birth-defect causing capabilities of LSD, but LSD has never conclusively been shown to cause birth deformities. An increased incidence of spontaneous abortions has been noted when pregnant women use LSD, but this is not too surprising since other ergot alkaloid derivatives are often used medically to induce labor and LSD shares this ability to a certain extent.

SUMMARY (LSD):

LSD is often viewed as the prototype for perceptual distorters. LSD and in general, the perceptual distorters, distort a persons perception of reality, causing a person, for instance to see sounds and hear colors. The drug effects are short lived but their use has been associated with becoming psychotic. There are many different drugs in this miscellaneous group which produce differing effects. Many people who use LSD or other perceptual distorters have enough of "bad trips" (poor experiences) and they "switch" to alcohol or pot and may become dependent on these drugs.

CHAPTER FIVE-B:

OTHER PERCEPTUAL DISTORTERS

1. PSILOCYBIN/PSILOCIN

The "sacred mushroom" has long been known by Mexican Indians to have hallucinogenic properties. The mushrooms used were probably of the genera Conocybe, Stropharia, and Psilocybe. The active agents in these mushrooms are psilocybin and its dephosphorylated derivative, psilocin. When ingested, the body rapidly dephosphorylates (removes a phosphate, or PO_4 group) the psilocybin molecules to form psilocin which apparently is the active form.

The major route of administration of psilocybin is oral and it is one of The most rapid acting of the hallucinogens by this route. Onset of actions occurs within 10 to 15 minutes and peak effects occur at about 90 minutes and do not start to subside until about 2 to 3 hours. Total duration of action is usually 5 to 6 hours, but this time may be increased with larger doses.

Physiologically and psychologically, psilocybin and LSD are very similar. Physical effects include the SNS stimulation causing increased heart rate, respiratory rate, increased body temperature, and dilated pupils. Psychic effects show increased sensory perception and vivid visual imagery. The major difference between LSD and psilocybin is that on a weight for weight basis, LSD is 150 to 200 times more potent. Therefore, 20mg of psilocybin is the dose required to obtain the same effects as 0.1mg of LSD.

Tolerance develops to the effects of psilocybin and cross-tolerance occurs with LSD and mescaline.

2. DMT (N,N DIMETHYLTRYPTAMINE)

DMT is the active substance isolated from the hallucinogenic snuff, cohoba, used by South American Indians. When taken orally, DMT is inactive so it must be inhaled as a powder or smoked in cigarettes, parsley, or marijuana which has been soaked in a DMT solution. Rarely is it injected.

DMT is chemically similar to psilocybin and both in turn, are derivatives of tryptamine. Tryptamine is a precursor (that is a substance from which another is derived) of the neurotransmitter serotonin, which many believe is the agent involved in much of the hallucinogenic activity. However, little or no cross tolerance exists between LSD and DMT so a different mechanism must also be involved.

The actions of LSD and DMT are very similar except that DMT has an extremely short duration of action. The effects of DMT will last only 30 to 60 minutes in the 30-40mg doses commonly used. Since the drug has very rapid onset of action, there may be little time for adjustment to the altered state of perception so that extreme panic reactions may be more common with DMT than with the other perceptual distorters. DMT, because of its very short action, has earned its slang name, the "business-man's lunch".

3. MORNING GLORY SEEDS/OLOLIUQUI

Ololiuqui is the Aztec name for the seeds of a wild, American morning glory species called Rivea corymbosa. When the seeds are eaten, effects of euphnoria, sedation, and hallucination are seen. The active ingredients in these seeds are lysergic acid derivatives, such as lysergic acid diethyl-amide. The potency of the seeds vary from batch to batch and so does the content of the other active ingredients in the seeds which might modu-late or modify the psychic as well as physical effects.

4. MESCALINE/PEYOTE

"Peyotyl" is the Aztec name given to the cactus, Lorphophora Williamsii, which grows in northern Mexico. The "buttons" or buds of this peyote cac-tus have been used for centuries in religious ceremonies and are still (legally) used today in the Native American Church of North America. Usually at least four peyote buttons are consumed during each ceremony. (Ceremonies last from sun down to sun up the next morning.) The active ingredient in the peyote cactus is mescaline, which has also been isolated from a number of other cactus varieties.

The actions of mescaline are very similar to those of LSD although the average doses are from 300 to 500mg, indicating that on a weight basis, LSD is approximately 1000 times as potent. When the entire peyote but-ton is ingested, instead of the purified mescaline, additional effects may be seen due to the presence of approximately fifteen other active agents.

The effects of mescaline are usually delayed with the appearance of nausea and vomiting being one of the first symptoms. The psychic phase does not start until about 1-2 hours after ingestion and it may persist for up to 12 hours. Visual imagery is prominent, but true hallucinations (where the user believes the images to be real) are rare. Little of the drug is metabolized with 60 to 90% excreted unchanged in the urine within 48 hours.

Mescaline is chemically similar to the drug amphetamine and also the naturally occurring neurotransmitters, epinephrine and norepinephrine. Mescaline use causes tolerance to develop as well as cross tolerance to LSD and psilocybin.

5. DOM (STP)

DOM (2,5-dimethoxy-4-methyl-amphetamine) is a term used synonomously with STP — "serenity, tranquility, peace". DOM is an amphetamine derivative which is also structurally similar to mescaline.

After oral intake, which is the usual route of use, effects appear in approximately 1 to 1 1/2 hours, reach a peak at about 3 to 4 hours and subside after 5 to 6 hours. Physical effects are similar to those seen with LSD and include increased salivation and tearing (a PSNS effect) as well as increased heart rate, blood pressure, respiration rate, and pupillary dilation (SNS effects). Psychic effects are also similar to LSD with vivid visual imagery and difficulty in controlling thoughts, expressions, and emotions. Tolerance does develop to DOM, but cross tolerance does not exist with LSD, mescaline or psilocybin. On a weight for weight basis, LSD is about 50 to 100 times more potent than DOM with a typical hallucinogenic dose of DOM being somewhere between 5 and 10mg orally.

6. MDA

MDA is an amphetamine derivative but possesses only mild SNS stimulating properties. The visual or auditory imagery associated with LSD is rarely found with MDA use. MDA produces a sense of physical well being, increased sensations of touch and, in some, an increased desire to be with other people. For this reason, it is sometimes referred to as the "love drug". Usually doses range from 100 to 150mg orally which makes LSD about 500 times more potent.

7. BELLADONNA ALKALOIDS

Four plants in the nightshade family have been associated with various religious rites as well as accidental and deliberate poisonings for hundreds of years. The plants are deadly nightshade (Atropa belladonna), jimson weed (Datura strommonium), henbane (Hyocyamus niger), and Angel's trumpet (Datura sauveolens).

The active constituents of these plants are atropine, scopolamine (hyoscine is the British equivalent of the term), and hyoscyamine. Collectively these compounds are referred to as the "belladonna alkaloids". Ingestion of any part of the plants or of the purified active ingredients will cause the production of a state which is closer to delirium than the psychic alterations produced by LSD. The mental symptoms seem to fall into two basic patterns. The person will either be wildly delirious, disoriented, restless and irritable with loud hallucinations; or stuporous, confused, uncoordinated, and unable to concentrate or respond appropriately. There is much more mental confusion and disorientation with the belladonna alkaloids, and in general, they produce a rather unpleasant trip.

The belladonna alkaloids are potent inhibitors of the neurotransmitter acetylcholine, so they are anticholinergics. Because of this, they cause a suppression of the PSNS (parasympathetic nervous system). The physical effects which occur will, therefore, not only represent a decreased PSNS effect, but also an increased SNS effect. As a matter-of-fact, the word Belladonna is a Latin word meaning "beautiful lady". The belladonna alkaloids were thought to give women beautiful, dark eyes (because they cause pupil dilation). Other symptoms could include a drying of all secretions, resulting in dry mouth and skin, flushing to compensate for decreased sweating, increased blood pressure heart rate and body temperature, urinary retention and constipation. The pupils will be dilated but close vision will be blurred. Some of the main differences between this syndrome and that seen with LSD use would be the hot, dry skin (as opposed to sweating), and an extreme amount of mental confusion. It has been said that the best description of belladonna use is that the person will be "dry as a bone, blind as a bat, red as a beet, and as mad as a hatter."

The belladonna alkaloids used to be found in many over-the-counter agents such as Compoz®, Quiet World®, Sleep-Eze®, and Sominex® since they also cause drowsiness, however in recent years, they have been replaced by antihistamines (such as Benadryl®), which are less dangerous. Besides this abundant availability of anticholinergic drugs, the nightshade plants grow wild throughout the country. Other anticolinergic compounds are synthesized to treat a wide variety of medical diseases (Parkinson's Disease, bladder dysfunctions, glaucoma, ulcers, etc.) and all of these synthetic agents can cause a belladonna-like syndrome if sufficient quantity is ingested. Some examples are trihexyphenidyl (Artane®) and benztropine (Cogentin®), two antiparkinsons drugs, both which have been used as perceptual distorters. Tolerance appears to develop to the actions of the belladonna and belladonna-like agents and cross tolerance appears within this group but not to any other of the hallucinogens. The mechanism of the psychic action of the belladonna alkaloids is not known but may be involved with the blocking of the neurotransmitter acetylcholine and its action in the brain.

SUMMARY (Miscellaneous Perceptual Distorters):

Just as is the case with LSD, these drugs all distort a persons perception of the world in which he or she lives by making them see sounds, hear colors, and walk out of high rise windows thinking they are leaving the house on the first floor. Although the end results of each drug may be the same, the mechanisms may differ, and often the peripheral effects differ from drug to drug in this class.

CHAPTER FIVE-C:

PHENCYCLIDINE (PCP)

1. INTRODUCTION

PCP was synthesized and tested in the 1950's as a general anesthetic. It proved to be very suitable as a pediatric anesthetic, however, on emergence from the anesthetized state, adult patients often exhibited extreme disorientation, agitation, and hallucinations. These symptoms were most often seen in young to middle aged male patients. Since 1965, PCP has (legally) only been available for use as an anesthetic in veterinary medicine. This is reflected in some of its street names (eg. Hog, Monkey, Tranq, Animal tranq).

2. BIOPHARMACEUTICS

PCP is highly lipid soluble and is absorbed well from any site. It is snorted, smoked, eaten and rarely, used intravenously. After smoking, the onset of action is within 2 to 5 minutes and peak blood levels occur at about 15 to 30 minutes. The duration of the intense action is approximately 4 to 6 hours, although it takes 24 to 48 hours for a complete return to "normal". It is fairly rapidly metabolized and excreted, so this long-term effect is not completely understood. It may be that the brain retains sufficient levels of PCP to have an effect long after blood levels have dropped. Man excretes a metabolite with no apparent psychic properties.

When PCP is eaten, it is absorbed from the small intestine, where it becomes more fat soluble. Onset of action after oral ingestion occurs within 15 minutes. Usually when PCP is taken by mouth, a greater amount is used than when it is smoked. This can lead to several problems since the duration of action depends on the dose taken. In other words, the greater the amount used, the longer PCP acts. A partial explanation of this is that with high doses, PCP is secreted back into the acid of the stomach (from the blood) since it is attracted to acid environments. When the PCP hits the alkaline conditions of the intestines, it is reabsorbed and can continue to cause an effect in the CNS. Spinal fluid is also slightly more acidic than blood so PCP is attracted there, too. Since the spinal fluid circulates through the brain, PCP gains access to and concentrates in the brain.

Phencylidine is mostly excreted in the urine and a great deal of unmetabolized drug appears. The urine, then, would be the optimal fluid for identification of PCP use. Urine tests are often positive for PCP up to seven days after ingestion.

3. PHARMACOLOGY

The mechanism of action of phencyclidine is unknown at this time. It somehow affects the flow of information coming into the brain which normally keeps the body informed as to what is going on around it, as well as, where the various body parts are in relationship to one another and to the environment. The body may appear to be several feet from the floor, or an arm or leg may appear foreign or unattached. The normal influx of sensory information seems to flood in and overload the brain to the point where a person cannot coherently grasp what is going on outside or inside the body. PCP appears to be unique in action compared with other perceptual distorting drugs and its effects are less dependent on the individual's personality than are the effects of LSD or mescaline.

Phencyclidine affects both sides of the autonomic nervous system, the SNS, and the PSNS. PCP stimulates the SNS so that tachycardia (rapid heart beat), increased blood pressure, and increased reflexes are seen. The PSNS is also stimulated by PCP so that sweating, drooling, and sometimes pupillary constriction occur.

The various signs and symptoms of PCP abuse are related to the amount used. At a low dose (1 to 5mg), the person may appear giddy and drunken, although marked anxiety and emotional outbursts are frequent. Staggering, slurred speech, tremulousness, numbness, and decreased pain sensitivity (especially of the face and neck) and muscle weakness may be present. There is also horizontal and vertical nystagmus (rapid, wandering movements of the pupils).

At a slightly higher dose (5-10mg), coma or stupor (often with the eyes open), increased blood pressure, shivering, muscle rigidity, vomiting, drooling, and distortion of body image may occur.

At high doses (greater than 10mg, usually taken orally), rigid arching of the back (the medical term for this is opisthotic posturing), seizuring, prolonged recovery marked by alternating periods of sleep and waking, perceptual distortions, disorientations and hallucinations may be present. Amnesia of these events usually follows, so the seriousness of the situation is not remembered at all by the user.

4. ADVERSE REACTIONS

Generally, most adverse reactions are likely to occur with doses greater than 10mg. The inexperienced user is much more likely to experience adverse effects since chronic users have learned to control their dosing through smoking. Since the onset with smoking is so rapid (2 to 5 minutes), the smoker can soon tell how "high" he is and determine whether to continue smoking or not. This dosing determination is very important since there is no standardization in the street-available preparations. In a study at The University of Southern California, there was a variation of PCP content from 0.1mg to 161.2mg per joint. Tablets, powder, and liquid preparations are also quite variable in their content and since their onset of action when taken orally is longer, it is hard to determine the dose until perhaps it is too late.

Quite a number of drug deaths have been reported due to PCP. Causes of death are status epilepticus (non-stop seizuring), cardiac or respiratory arrest, or a hypertensive crisis (where the blood pressure is extemely elevated) which can cause rupture of blood vessels in the brain. Deaths can occur even when PCP blood levels have dropped back to zero.

Deaths also occur with PCP abuse due to "behavioral toxicity". This term denotes the fact that people who are high on PCP often cannot correlate events occurring in their environment. Thus, in an emergency situation, they are unable to correctly react. Drownings may occur, also a person on PCP may not be able to flee from fire or other dangers such as moving vehicles.

PSYCHOSIS

Psychosis is an all too common occurrence after PCP use. It usually comes after the use of very high doses or after prolonged coma. In one study done by the military, there were 9 patients admitted to a hospital with PCP-induced psychoses. The duration of the psychosis ranged from 6 to 90 days, and one patient was still not improved after 90 days. The psychosis appears to resolve spontaneously and the usual antipsychotic medications have little or no effect on the condition. The prolonged effect does not seem to be limited to people with pre-existing psychosis.

MUSCLE DAMAGE

When a person on PCP becomes violent, the use of restraints may become necessary. If the person fights the restraints, muscle damage can occur. The dead muscle tissue will then slough off into the blood stream. During kidney filtration of the blood, pieces of the dead tissue will clog up the kidney and if sufficient damage occurs, kidney failure and possible death can result.

5. TOLERANCE

Evidence of tolerance or a withdrawal syndrome is incomplete, although some users report psychological dependence and tolerance to the psychic effects of PCP.

6. CHRONIC USE

Following periods of prolonged PCP use, paranoia, auditory hallucinations, violent behavior, anxiety, and severe depression can occur. Massive oral overdoses are seen most frequently in the chronic user who is depressed and in possession of large amounts of PCP. It is usually ingested in a suicide attempt. These people may also become involved in unusual car accidents or criminal behavior.

Chronic users can also develop an organic brain dysfunction which continues long after the cessation of PCP use. These people have memory gaps, some disorientation, perhaps visual disturbances and they commonly have difficulty with speech. The latter problem may be due to an inability to recall the proper words. The condition may improve with discontinuation of PCP use.

7. CONTAMINANTS/DERIVATIVES

As if all these problems were not enough with PCP, there is a contaminant that has been found in certain PCP batches called PCC (l-piperidine-cyclohexanecarbonile). PCC is also strongly psychoactive and there is a high incidence of nausea, bloody vomiting, abdominal cramping, and several deaths have been reported. PCC is an unstable compound and one of its breakdown products is piperidine which has a "fishy" odor. A batch of PCP with a fishy odor is more than likely contaminated with PCC.

TCP is a derivative of PCP. It is an acceptable substitute to PCP users since it has similar, if not stronger, effects. There are also approximately 30 other chemical derivatives of PCP which are similar and easily manufactured. TCP has been made illegal, but legislation is having a hard time keeping up with all the new derivatives.

Ketamine is an approved and used anesthetic agent which is similar to PCP. It is called a "dissociative anesthetic" since patients are somewhat conscious but are dissociated from their surrounding environment during surgery. Twelve percent of all the patients who have been given ketamine experience some sort of psychological manifestations which vary between dream-like states, vivid imagery, hallucinations, and emergency delirium. These adverse effects have not been seen in pediatric patients, possibly due to a different metabolism, so the use of ketamine has basically been limited to children.

SUMMARY (PCP):

In small dosages PCP acts like a mild sedative drug. In increasing dosages it tends to have greater anesthetic-like properties and in large quantities patients tend to become depersonalized, hostile, and violent.

CHAPTER 6

Marijuana

CHAPTER SIX:

MARIJUANA

1. INTRODUCTION

Marijuana is the term used to denote the leaves and flowering tops of the plant Cannibis sativa. The various preparations of Cannibis sativa constitute the most widely used illicit drug in the world.

CHEMISTRY

The main psychoactive ingredient in marijuana is delta-9-tetrahydro-cannabinol, also called delta-9-THC or just THC for short. THC content in marijuana varies from plant to plant due to genetic and environmental factors. The THC content of most marijuana sold in the U.S. ranges from 0.9% to 1.0%. There is practically no THC found in the stems, roots or seeds of the plant. It is basically present only in the leaves and flowering parts. More potent preparations can be made of cannibis by using just the flowering parts of the plant. The most potent preparation of cannibis is made when the resinous exudate of the flower is collected. This product is called hashish or "hash" and the THC content ranges from 5 to 15%. Pure THC can be made synthetically, but the cost is prohibitive.

One of the complicating factors in the study of marijuana is that THC is not the only component. Besides THC, marijuana contains several dozen other compounds, which are chemically classed as cannabinoids, terpenes, and sterols. Also, each sample tends to be slightly different from the others. How these compounds interact and modify the actions of each other still remains to be fully explored. This discussion will basically be about the actions of delta-9-THC, since more is known about it than any other component of marijuana.

EPIDEMIOLOGY

Several studies indicate that about one half of all people who try marijuana experimentally continue to use it. More importantly, it is estimated that more than 50 million Americans have tried marijuana. Also of interest are the following estimates:

—59.5% of the high school seniors graduating in 1981 had used marijuana at least once. (This count excluded drop-outs who have an even higher rate of use.)

—34% of the high school seniors graduating in 1981 began smoking marijuana before entering high school.

In the past two decades, there has been a striking increase in marijuana use.

—In 1962, 4% of persons between the ages of 18 and 25 years had ever used marijuana.
—In 1971, 39% of persons between the ages of 18 and 25 years had ever used marijuana.
—In 1980, 68% of persons between the ages of 18 and 25 years had ever used marijuana.

MEDICAL USES

There have been several experimental medical uses for delta-9-THC, and investigation has been ongoing to develop synthetic derivatives of it which are devoid of psychoactivity, yet can be medically useful. The suggested medical uses of delta-9-THC include the following:

Glaucoma: THC can lower pressure within the eye and has been seen to be effective in certain cases of glaucoma.

Asthma: THC causes dilation of the airways and has been used for centuries in primitive cultures to treat asthma. However, the smoke from marijuana is irritating to the airways and is not a good means of delivering the THC to the lungs.

Epilepsy: THC causes an increase in electrical thresholds of brain cells so it may be useful in treating seizure disorders.

Nausea and vomiting: The metabolite of THC called C-THC is probably the compound which suppresses nausea and vomiting. This can be very useful in the treatment of cancer patients in whom nausea and vomiting are frequent side effects of their radiation and chemotherapeuatic treatments.

2. BIOPHARMACEUTICS

Marijuana is commonly smoked in cigarette form, called a joint. With smoking, less than 50% of the THC is absorbed and enters the circulation, the rest is lost by inappropriate inhalation or accumulation in the lung tissue. The onset of action, when smoked, is within minutes. Peak effects occur at 20 to 30 minutes, and the action ceases between 1 and 2 hours.

Marijuana can also be ingested (taken orally) and is usually cooked up in some type of preparation, such as brownies or cookies. After ingestion, onset of action occurs in about one hour, peak effects occur in about 4 to 5 hours. With ingestion: about 95% of the THC is absorbed, however, since it is absorbed over a much long period of time, blood level peaks will only be 1/3 to 1/2 as high as those achieved by smoking an equivalent amount.

THC is very fat soluble. After being absorbed, it rapidly leaves the blood, and is well distributed to body organs and especially concentrating in fat tissue. THC remains in the brain, reproductive organs, and in fat tissue for relatively long periods of time because it undergoes no breakdown in these tissues, but must pass back into the blood and reach the liver to be metabolized. The T 1/2 of marijuana in fat tissue is 8 days.

Because THC is highly lipid soluble, the liver must metabolize it to more water soluble compounds so that it can be excreted. One metabolite is 11-hydroxy-delta 9-THC which is also active. Another metabolite of THC is 11-nor-9-carboxy-delta 9-THC (C-THC). C-THC appears within minutes after smoking and is measurable in the blood long after delta 9-THC disappears. C-THC could account for the anti-nauseant effect of marijuana. It is long lasting and is now being explored for use in cancer patients on chemotherapy.

THC disappears rapidly from the blood and is stored in the fatty tissues of the body. From the fat tissues, excretion progresses slowly with only 60% of a dose showing up in the urine and 20% in the bile after one week. THC metabolism is increased with chronic use so that the T 1/2 for chronic smokers is about 27 hours compared to a T 1/2 of 56 hours in nonsmokers. This enzyme induction will then overcome the tendency to get too much of a build-up of the THC in the fatty tissues.

3. PHARMACOLOGY

The psychopharmacology of marijuana is very complex and marijuana does not fit into a class with any of the other psychoactive drugs. At low doses, marijuana has almost a stimulant effect with mild euphoria, increased sensory awareness and appreciation and alterations in time perception. With increasing doses, a sedative-like effect occurs characterized by impaired short-term memory, lapses of attention, disturbed thought patterns and passivity. With very high doses, there are changes in body image, depersonalization, and marked sensory distortion which are similar to effects seen with LSD and mescaline. Thus, the effects of marijuana are, to a great extent, dose dependent. The very high dose effects are rarely seen in the U.S. since the THC content here is usually lower. These effects have been seen in India where hash eating is common and the THC content in all marijuana preparations is quite high.

The physical changes which accompany marijuana use are more well defined and easier to observe than the psychological changes. Tachycardia (accelerated heart beat) is very prominent, although the exact mechanism by which it occurs is not known. ECG (electrocardiogram) changes have also been seen with marijuana use, with the greatest changes occurring in chronic users. There is a possibility, then, that long-term use of marijuana actually damages the heart muscle. This area needs further research though, before conclusions can be drawn.

High doses of marijuana also affects the blood pressure by causing postural hypotension. This means that if a person stands up too fast, they could faint since the blood pressure is reduced and there may be a decrease in the amount of blood getting up to the brain. Since marijuana can cause hypotension, it must have some effect on dilating the blood vessels of the body. This effect is most visible in the conjunctiva (the "whites" of the eyes) regardless of whether marijuana is smoked or ingested. The blood vessels of the conjunctiva will be dilated and the eyes will look very red. The eyes may also feel dry due to a decrease in tear production. There is also a decrease in salivary flow which results in a condition referred to by users as "cotton mouth".

Marijuana has been observed to increase the appetite for sweets in some users even though chronic marijuana use can cause glucose intolerance. In fact, with acute marijuana intoxication a person taking a glucose tolerance test would appear to be diabetic. The insulin present in the blood is still there in normal amounts. However, marijuana stimulates the release of a compound called growth hormone which works against insulin and causes the blood glucose levels to remain elevated.

One last effect of marijuana is that like the sedative-hypnotics, it causes a suppression of REM sleep and REM rebound can occur with cessation of use. The REM rebound from marijuana may last months and be characterized by recurrent nightmares.

4. ADVERSE REACTIONS

NAUSEA AND VOMITING: The most frequent adverse reactions encountered with marijuana are nausea, vomiting and dizziness. This may be due somewhat to smoke poisoning, but may also be a direct, early effect of THC.

BRONCHITIS: Frequent use of marijuana cigarettes may produce bronchitis, asthma, sinusitis, or chronic redness of the eyes because of an irritant effect.

IMPAIRED IMMUNITY: Under certain conditions, marijuana impairs a component of the white blood cell defense system. This work was all done as test tube research. However, more clinical data needs to be collected before it is determined if marijuana increases the susceptibility to infections or tumors.

BIRTH DEFECTS: THC has not been shown to cause birth defects. However, studies have not been undertaken with the other compounds in marijuana.

CANCER: It has been speculated that smoke from marijuana, like tobacco smoke, accelerates malignant cell transformation of lung cells to cause cancer.

AMOTIVATIONAL SYNDROME: An "amotivational syndrome" has been described in certain marijuana users who lose interest in their jobs, school, family, etc. However, the exact role of marijuana in this condition is unclear.

PSYCHOSIS: Drug psychosis has been seen with acute intoxication. This is characterized by confusion, delusions, hallucinations, emotional instability, excitement, disorientation, depersonalization, paranoid symptoms and temporary amnesia. This is mostly seen only in India where the marjuana is much more potent. Often, the people who are afflicted with this condition have some sort of predisposing factors such as severe stress, a family history of schizophrenia or some pre-existing psychological problem. The psychosis will usually disappear when marijuana usage is stopped.

STERILITY: Clinical symptoms from chronic and continuous use of marijuana are only recently becoming apparent, because regular or frequet long term use of the drug has been a recent occurence in the Western world. One of the areas of study in chronic effects of THC has been the reproductive organs. There is evidence indicating that prolonged, intense marijuana use can cause abnormal sperm, as well as reduced sperm count, and decreased sperm motility in humans.

Chronic use of marijuana is associated with disruption of the menstrual cycle in some cases.

TOLERANCE AND WITHDRAWAL: In experimental studies in the U.S. where extremely high doses of THC have been used, and occurrence of tolerance has been observed. The withdrawal period was then characterized by sleep disturbances, irritability, restlessness, decreased appetite, sweating and sudden weight loss due to previous fluid retention.

SUMMARY (Marijuana)

—The active marijuana ingredient is delta 9-THC.
—It is most commonly smoked as a joint.
—Delta 9-THC remains in fat tissue for extended periods, but its activity is not known.
—THC effects vary with dosage:
  —low dosage causes euphoric and some stimulant effects.
  —increasing dosages result in sedative effects.
  —high doses cause depersonalization and sensory disturbances.
—Chronic usage is associated with an amotivational syndrome.
—Withdrawal may occur with chronic usage.

Perhaps no other psychoactive drug evokes such controversy as marijuana. Most people smoke pot in this country and there is a lack of scientific information regarding its real effect. Many people use marijuana with other psychoactive drugs and see no reason to stop. Although each case needs to be evaluated individually there seems to be a tendency for people who are chemically dependent or addicted to get into more trouble if they continue using marijuana. And it should be noted that more and more, patients are asking for help in getting off marijuana.

CHAPTER 7

Inhalants

CHAPTER SEVEN:

INHALANTS

The inhalants are volatile substances (chemicals which are vaporized to a gaseous form at normal room temperature) which are introduced into the body via the lungs. This method of administration provides rapid on-set of intoxication and easy access.

The inhalants can be divided into three loose categories:

(1) the anesthetics such as ether and nitrous oxide,
(2) the volatile, commercial solvents such as benzene, toluene, gasoline, etc., and
(3) the vasodilating nitrites such as amyl and isobutyl nitrite.

Since there are certain basic differences in the groups, each will be covered separately.

1. ANESTHETICS

Long before their anesthetic properties were utilized in medicine, ether, chloroform, and nitrous oxide ("laughing gas") were used by lay people to become intoxicated. Ether can be taken by mouth, but the most usual method of administration of these substances is inhalation. Since these substances are anesthetics, it would be beneficial to review the stages of anesthesia. Stage I is the induction phase and is characterized by a generalized neurological and physical depression, possibly accompanied by euphoria. Stage II is excitatory and slurred speech, hallucinations, irritability, vomiting, shouting, etc., can occur. This appears to be caused by the depression of normal inhibitory functions, somewhat in the manner that the depressant, alcohol, causes a "stimulatory" effect due to the loss of inhibitions. Stage III is where anesthesia occurs. Stage IV is accompanied by respiratory arrest which is fatal if respiration is not assisted, and Stage V is where cardiac arrest occurs and death will result.

Within this category, the most common anesthetic which is used to obtain a "high" is nitrous oxide. This gas is relatively nontoxic and death, if it occurs, is usually due to asphyxiation, from an over usage of the nitrous oxide resulting in inadequate oxygen intake. Since the gas is inhaled, absorption through the pulmonary membranes is rapid so that effects are felt almost immediately but the duration of action is short, since it is re-expired via the lungs and little metabolism occurs.

Halothane (Fluothane), is a recently synthesized anesthetic agent. It is also increasing in abuse potential due to its easy availability in hospitals. Halothane is a fluorinated, chlorinated compound. Compounds containing fluorine and chlorine are usually quite toxic to the liver. Little is known, however, concerning the long term effects of intermittent usage of these substances.

2. COMMERCIAL SOLVENTS

Commercial solvents are those products which are used in such preparations as lacquers, paints, glues, cleaners, etc. These compounds are highly volatile. This means that they evaporate easily to produce fumes by a variety of means; from a handkerchief, from a small plastic bag, or even from a plastic bag placed over the head or body. Obviously, the use of these solvents in a confined place can lead to a lack of oxygen and death could occur from asphyxiation.

STRAIGHT-CHAINED HYDROCARBONS are also called aliphatic hydrocarbons. The prototype of the straight-chained hydrocarbons to be considered here is hexane. Hexane is found in many glues and in plastic cement.

Biopharmaceutics

Hexane is lipid soluble so it readily crosses membrane barriers in the lung and enters the blood stream without passing through the liver. It is not metabolized to any great extent before it reaches the CNS. With the rapid absorption and minimal early metabolism, the onset of action is very fast and somewhat intense, but of short duration.

Like all lipid soluble compounds, hexane gains rapid entry into the brain and all fatty tissues.

Hexane is metabolized in the liver by microsomal enzyme systems to more water soluble products by the addition of oxygen and -OH groups. Two products of metabolism may be the causitive agents in the neurotoxicity (nerve damage) seen with hexane use. Excretion of these metabolites is partly through the urine and partially via expired air.

Pharmacology

Just as with the anesthetics, the main action of all of the commercial volatile solvents is depressive. Generalized depression is the first effect seen and depression of inhibitory functions causes the excitation and stimulation which might occur. Slurred speech, staggering gait, mental confusion, and emotional instability are seen which are all very similar to the signs and symptoms typical of alcohol intoxication. As the state deepens, drowsiness will occur and increase to stupor or coma in high doses.

Little has been done to determine the toxic effects of solvent use. Death with hexane has been known to occur. These deaths are usually very sudden and appear to be due to fatal cardiac arrhythmias (loss of normal rhythm. In animal studies, it appears that all the solvents can somehow make the heart more sensitive to epinephrine (adrenalin). In this state, any epinephrine stimulation, for instance fear, can cause the heart rhythm to be seriously disrupted. Death can also occur due to respiratory depression in high doses.

Hexane has also been shown to cause a breakdown in peripheral nerve fibers, resulting in numbness, tremor, etc. This process appears to be due to the metabolites of hexane and improvement usually occurs when usage is stopped.

As with all of the commercial solvents, tolerance can develop to the CNS effects of hexane. Psychological dependence can also occur but as yet no well defined physical dependence or withdrawal has been documented with solvent use.

Gasoline, another straight-chained hydrocarbon, is used in many rural and isolated areas, especially where alcohol is not available. Gasoline has a number of toxic potentials due to all of the additives in it. Triorthocryesyl has been shown to cause spastic muscle wasting diseases, while lead additives can cause acute and chronic brain damage. Benzene is also found in gasoline and it is associated with a number of blood disorders.

This problem of combination products is almost universal among the commercial preparations since they are rarely one pure compound. Thus, the toxic effects will always be a combination of the toxicology of the individual agents, making an accurate diagnosis of solvent abuse difficult since the pharmacologic picture may be confusing.

CYCLIC HYDROCARBONS are also called aromatic hydrocarbons. These hydrogen and carbon compounds are in ring structure arrangements and the prototype for this group is benzene. Benzene is found in many plastic cements, lacquers, paint remover, gasoline, and cleaning fluids. This group also contains toluene, xylene, naphthalene, and many others.

Biopharmaceutics

Benzene, like all of the commercial solvents, is very lipid soluble and readily passes through the membranes in the lung to enter the blood circulation. It is distributed throughout the body in fatty tissues such as the brain. Due to the rapid absorption, onset of action is also very rapid and the duration of effects is short, being only about 1/2 to 1 hour.

Pharmacology

The pharmacology of benzene is basically the same as that of hexane. Benzene is a depressant and intoxication greatly resembles intoxication with alcohol. However, the toxic problems with the cyclic hydrocarbons are slightly different than those seen with the straight-chained hydrocarbons. One of the biggest problems with benzene and the other cyclic hydrocarbons is their suppression of bone marrow, which is where the components of blood are formed. This results in anemia (decreased red blood cells), leukopenia (decreased white blood cells), or thrombocytopenia (decreased platelets, one of the elements necessary for clot formation). If all occur simultaneously, it is called pancytopenia. The cause of this toxic problem may be that the metabolites of compounds bind with cells in the bone marrow and cause a breakdown in the normal manufacture of the blood components. The cyclic hydrocarbons can cause death and it appears to be due to cardiac arrhythmias and respiratory depression which also occurs with the straight-chained hydrocarbons.

CHLORINATED HYDROCARBONS are the most frequently encountered substances in this group, and carbon tetrachloride, which is used in spot removing and other cleaning substances is the most commonly abused chlorinated hydrocarbon.

Biopharmaceutics

Carbon tetrachloride is lipid soluble, so it is rapidly absorbed and distributed to fatty tissue, such as the brain. It is predominantly excreted unmetabolized via the lungs with a small percent excreted in the urine. Carbon tetrachloride is excreted very slowly over a 2 to 3 month period, so chronic use can lead to seriously high concentrations in the body and chronic intoxication.

Pharmacology

The basic effect of carbon tetrachloride is that of a depressant, but it also has certain highly dangerous toxic effects. Carbon tetrachloride may cause a number of gastrointestinal symptoms including nausea, vomiting, loss of appetite, abdominal pain, and loss of weight. Chlorinated compounds can be very toxic to the liver and kidneys and if the damage is severe enough, death can result from liver and kidney failure. Once again, sudden death can occur from cardiac arrhythmias, and respiratory depression results with high doses.

FREONS are chlorinated, fluorinated compounds used as propellants in aerosals and coolants in refrigeration systems.

Biopharmaceutics

The freons are lipid soluble, and are therefore rapidly absorbed and distributed to fatty tissues such as the brain. Little is known, however, concerning their metabolism and excretion.

Pharmacology

The pharmacology of the freons is similar to that of other commercial solvents. Although these compounds contain chlorine and fluorine groups, little liver or kidney damage has been attributed to their usage. However, this may be due to lack of toxicologic capabilities. Freon use has been documented to cause sudden death from cardiac arrhythmias and the use of freons carry other hazards as well. When use in the aeresol form, airway freezing can occur due to the rapid evaporation of freon from the airway linings. Spasm of the airway may cause it to shut and this can obviously lead to trouble. Also, with the use of aerosols, there is the risk that the active agent of the spray (i.e. deodorant, paint, etc.) can cause much damage of its own. Luckily, the use of freons has been greatly restricted by the U.S. government due to the damaging effects the freons have on the ozone layer of the atmosphere. However, freons are still available in many medical aerosols and are still sold as refrigerants.

3. NITRITES

The classic example of the nitrite group is amyl nitrite, also known as isoamyl nitrite. The tradenames for this compound include Vaprole® and Aspirole®. Amyl nitrite is available only on prescription and is supplied in small, crushable ampules which contain 0.3ml of the compound.

Another drug, isobutyl (or just butyl) nitrite has made its way into products available at many "head-shops" and adult book stores under such names as "Locker Room", "Rush", "Kick", "Jock Aroma", etc. Both compounds are quite similar in action, so amyl nitrite will be used as the example here.

Biopharmaceutics

Amyl nitrite is rapidly absorbed through the membranes of the lungs into the blood stream and it crosses the blood brain barrier easily. It has an onset of action within 2-3 minutes and a duration of only about 15 to 20 minutes. It is rapidly broken down by the liver and is excreted via the expired air and the urine.

Pharmacology

The nitrites are potent vasodilators and are used medically for acute angina attacks. Angina is a disease characterized by heart pains which occur upon exertion in people whose hearts don't pump well. When all the blood vessels are dilated, there is less resistance to the pumping of the heart, so not as much energy is needed and the pain of angina stops. Amyl nitrite is one of the few inhalants frequently used by adults and it is due to the claim of sexual enhancement. The apparent effect is a lengthening of time and intensity of orgasm, possibly due to a dilation of genital arteries. Also, there appears to be a decrease in blood flow in cerebral arteries which could cause dizziness and euphoria possibly contributing to the sexual intensification.

Other actions caused by amyl nitrite are, increased heart rate due to the vasodilation, and increased blood flow back to the heart. Also due to the vasodilation, extreme flushing may be present as well as a pounding headache. Nausea, dizziness and weakness may also occur.

With regular usage, tolerance to the effects of the nitrites can occur, but a withdrawal syndrome has never been reported.

The main difference with butyl nitrite is that it is not absorbed quite as fast as amyl nitrite, so blood levels of the drug do not rise as high, and the duration of action is somewhat longer, but the effects are less intense.

SUMMARY (Inhalants)

—There are three categories of inhalants:
  (1) anesthetic
  (2) volatile solvents
  (3) vasodilating nitrites
—Anesthetics are drugs which put people to sleep, for example, nitrous oxide and chloroform.
—Volatile solvents are drugs which are easily changed from liquids to vapors such as gases or glues.
—Nitrites are drugs which dilate blood vessels such as amyl nitrite. They are abused as aphrodisiac agents.

Inhalants are primarily used by young people who are less than 18 years old. The trend of solvent usage has expanded to include paints, glues, nail polish removers, gasoline, liquid paper, etc. The effects of solvents are about the same as for sedative hypnotics and many young people who used inhalants may end up dependent on alcohol or other sedative type drugs.

APPENDIXES

APPENDIX A

Included here are some of the chemical structures and many of the major chemical reactions of the drugs and classes of drugs discussed in the chapters.

1. ALCOHOL is covered in Chapter 2A. The major reactions and structures are included in the biopharmaceutics and pharmacology sections.

2. BARBITURATES are covered in Chapter 2B. The basic chemical structure of the barbiturates is:

The positions marked R_1, R_2, R_3, and X are variable positions. Various substitutions at these positions change the biopharmaceutic properties. The R_1, and R_2, side chains determine the lipid solubility — as chain length and branching increases, so does lipid solubility.

The most important route of bariturate metabolism is hydroxylation (addition of an -OH group) of the R_1 and R_2 chains.

3. BENZODIAZEPINES are covered in Chapter 2C. Some typical benzodiazepine structures are:

CHLORDIAZEPOXIDE   DIAZEPAM   ELURAZEPAM

You may recall from the chapter that most of the benzodiazepines have at least one active metabolite. Note the metabolism of diazepam:

DIAZEPAM   NOR-DIAZEPAM (ACTIVE)   OXAZEPAM (ACTIVE)   GLUCURONIDE RAPIDLY EXCRETED

Following is a summary of benzodiazepines and their major active metabolites.

GENERIC NAME	TRADE NAME	ACTIVE METABOLITES
diazepam	Valium®	desmethyldiazepam (T 1/2=30-60 hrs)
chlordiazepoxide	Librium®	many
clorazepate	Tranxene®	desmethyldiazepam
prazepam	Centrax/Verstran®	3-OH prazepam desmethyldiazepam
flurazepam	Dalmanė®	desalkylflurazepam (T 1/2=50-100 hrs)
halazepam	Poxipam®	n-3-OH halazepam desmethyldiazepam
oxazepam	Serax®	none
alprazolam	Xanax®	alpha-OH alprazolam
temazepam	Restoril®	insignificant
triazolam	Halcion®	-OH triazolan
clonazepam	Clonipin®	several
lorazepam	Ativan®	none

4. OTHER (MISCELLANEOUS) SEDATIVE HYPNOTIC DRUGS were discussed in Chapter 2D.

a. Meprobamate:

b. Methyprylon:

c. Glutethimide:

d. Ethchlorvynol:

e. Chloral hydrate (included is the active metabolite trichloroethanol, and the major metabolic reactions.)

f. Methaqualone:

5. NARCOTIC ANALGESICS AND NARCOTIC ANTAGONISTS were covered in chapter 3. Below are some representatives of the class:

AGONISTS:

Morphine

Methadone

Meperidine

ANTAGONIST:

Naloxone

AGONIST ANTAGONIST:

Pentazocine

Heroin is made by adding two -COCH$_3$ chemcial groups at certain positions on the morphine molecule.

The metabolism of narcotic analgesics is very complicated. (If you question this, just look at the flow chart on the next page.) Many processes of metabolism are involved, but only the four most important, N-dealkylation, O-dealkylation, hydrolysis, and conjugation, will be discussed here.

1. N-dealkylation means that the CH3 (or other similar groups) attached to the nitrogen atom on the molecule is "chopped" off. (See diagram on next page.) When the group attached to the N is only a -CH3, N-dealkylation is called N-demethylation, because a CH3 is also called a methyl group. When N-demethylation occurs to morphine, codeine, meperidine, or methadone, the resultant metabolite is normorphine, norcodeine, etc. This is an important pathway for meperidine (33%), but less important for morphine (1-5%) and codeine (10%). Norcodeine is as potent an analgesic as codeine, however, the potency of normorphine and normeperidine is decreased, while the toxicity is increased. Methadone, and the investigational drug LAAM are also converted to active "nor-" metabolites, which account for their longer durations of action.

2. O-dealkylation, or O-demethylation means "chopping off" a -CH3 or similar group from an oxygen (O) atom. The most important example of this type of metabolism is the conversion of codeine to morphine via O-demethylation. This accounts for 10% of codeine metabolism.

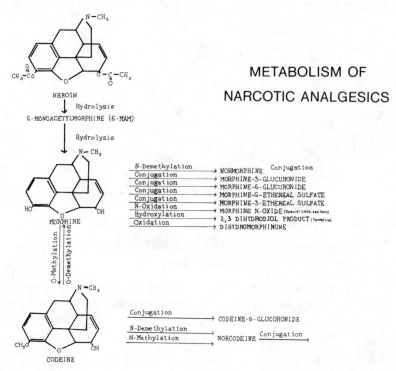

METABOLISM OF

NARCOTIC ANALGESICS

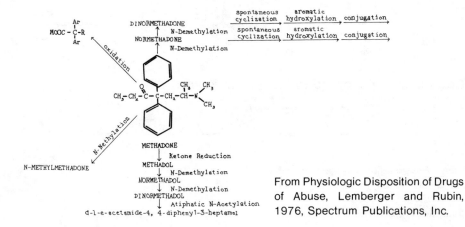

From Physiologic Disposition of Drugs of Abuse, Lemberger and Rubin, 1976, Spectrum Publications, Inc.

3. Hydrolysis is a metabolic process which uses hydrogen atoms and oxygen atoms in the same ratio as water (H_2O) in order to split large molecules into smaller ones. (An example of this is at the right.) An acetyl group, CH3-C=0, is split off of the heroin molecule, and an H atom is added in its place, while an -OH is added to the acetyl group. (H + OH = H_2O... water!) Hydrolysis of narcotic analgesics occurs mainly in the liver, but large quantities of the necessary enzymes also are present in the brain, serum, and kidneys, and some hydrolysis occurs at these locations. The hydrolysis of heroin first results in formation of 6-MAM, which is an active metabolite and eventually in formation of morphine. Hydrolysis is also the major pathway of metabolism of meperidine.

HEROIN

Hydrolysis

G-MONOACETYLMORPHINE (G-MAM)
+
CH₃-COH

4.   Conjugation is the combining of a drug molecule with either glucuronic acid (to form glucuronides) or sulfuric acid (to form sulfates) making a more water soluble molecule which can not cross the BBB and which is easily excreted via the kidneys. The conjugate is the final metabolic product of morphine, codeine, heroin, and most of the other narcotic analgesics.

6.   Psychomotor stimulants were discussed in Chapter 4. These are their structures:

AMPHETAMINE

METHYLPHENIDATE

COCAINE

Cocaine is metabolized to inactive products.

COCAINE   BENZOYLECGONINE   + CH₃ OH   ECGONINE
                                         METHANOL
                                                                    BENZOIC ACID

From Physiologic Disposition of Drugs of Abuse. Lemberger and Rubin, 1976.
Spectrum Publications, Inc.

There are active metabolites of the amphetamines (review metabolism section in Chapter 4, of amphetamines), however, methylphenidate has none.

METHYLPHENIDATE   RITALINIC ACID

From
Physiologic Disposition of Drugs
of Abuse, Lemberger and Rubin,
1976, Spectrum Publications, Inc.

7. The structures of the major perceptual distorters are:

8. The major active ingredient in marijuana is delta-9-THC:

APPENDIX B: GLOSSARY

ABSORPTION:
Process of a drug gaining entry into the main circulation.

ABSTINENCE:
Discontinuence and avoidance of further use of a drug of dependency by a drug dependent person.

ACETALDEHYDE:
Toxic substance which is the product of the first step in metabolism of alcohol.

ACNE ROSACEA:
Redness and swelling of the nose and cheeks which is often seen in long term alcohol dependent persons.

ADDICTION (DRUG):
A state of periodic or chronic intoxication, detrimental to the individual and society, produced by repeated consumption of the drug, and characterized by a compulsion to take the drug, a tendency to increase the amount consumed, and withdrawal upon cessation of drug use.

ADDITIVE EFFECTS:
The enhancement of the effect of one chemical by the presence of another. The effect is doubled or equal to the combined amount of the two chemicals.

AFFECTIVE (NERVE TRANSMISSION):
Messages coming into the brain.

AGONIST:
A chemical which stimulates a response at a cell receptor site.

ALCOHOL DEHYDROGENASE:
A liver enzyme involved in the reaction which converts alcohol to acetaldehyde.

ANALGESIC:
Pain reliever.

ANESTHETIC:
A substance which causes loss of consciousness and insensibility to pain. (A local anesthetic causes loss of sensation to localized area.)

ANTAGONIST:
A chemical which opposes or impedes action of another.

ANTICHOLINERGIC EFFECTS:
Antagonistic to the action of parasympathetic or other cholinergic nerve fibers.

AUTONOMIC NERVOUS SYSTEM:
System of nerves controlling many internal processes, such as heart rate, digestive processes, pupil diameter, etc.

BENZODIAZEPINE:
The chemical class of sedative hypnotic drugs which includes drugs similar to diazepam, lorazepam, and chlordiazepoxide, etc.

BIOPHARMACEUTICS:
How the body processes a drug.

BIPHASIC (HALF-LIFE):
The type of drug half-life which is marked by two distinctly different rates of clearance from the blood.

BLOOD BRAIN BARRIER:
The lipid membranes which impede transfer of many substances from the blood stream into brain tissue.

CANNABINOID:
A derivative or preparation from the plant cannibis sativa, containing the ingredient delta-9-tetrahydrocannabinol.

CATALASE SYSTEM:
One pathway of ethanol metabolism, involving use of hydrogen peroxide.

CATALYST:
A substance that increases the rate of chemical reaction.

CENTRAL NERVOUS SYSTEM (CNS):
The nerves which make up the brain and spinal cord.

CHEMICAL:
Substance capable of altering body function.

CHLORINATED:
Addition of a chlorine atom to a basic molecular structure.

CHOLINERGIC EFFECTS:
Effects similar to those induced by acetylcholine. These are the type seen with stimulation of parasympathetic nervous system.

CIRRHOSIS:
A chronic liver disease marked by scarring of liver tissue and eventually liver failure.

CONFABULATION:
The inventing of tales and readiness to produce fluent answers without regard to facts, to any question put.

CONJUGATION:
In metabolism of chemicals, the combination (usually in the liver) of the chemical with glucuronic acid or sulfuric acid to form a more water soluble compound for excretion.

CROSS TOLERANCE:
A diminished or reduced response to the effects of a psychoactive chemical due to the prior use of another psychoactive chemical. True cross tolerance is confined to drugs in the same pharmacological class.

CYCLIC HYDROCARBON:
Chemicals composed of hydrogen and carbon which exist in ring form.

CYTOPLASM:
The fluid and structures within a cell wall and surrounding the cell nucleus.

DEMENTIA:
A mental deterioration due to organic or emotional causes.

DEPENDENCY:
Psychic or physical state resulting from the interaction between a living organism and a psychoactive drug characterized by behavioral and other responses that always include a compulsion to take the drug on a continuous or periodic basis in order to experience its psychic effects and sometimes avoid the discomfort of its abstinence.

DISTRIBUTION:
The pattern of specific organs or areas of the body to which the drug spreads or concentrates.

DISULFIRAM ETHANOL REACTION:
The group of symptoms which are seen as a result of blocking the metabolism of acetaldehyde.

DIURESIS:
Urine excretion in excess of the usual amount.

DRUG:
A substance with potential use as medicine in treatment of disease.

DYSPHORIA:
A feeling of being ill at ease.

ENTEROHEPATIC CIRCULATION:
The blood transport system which runs between the intestines and the liver.

ENZYME INDUCTION:
Increase in ability to metabolize a drug(s) or endogenous substance(s) due to increased activity of specific metabolic enzymatic systems caused by previous substance administration.

ENZYME:
Protein molecules which act as catalysts in biochemical reactions.

ETHANOL:
Ethyl alcohol; or the beverage type of alcohol.

EUPHORIA:
The extreme sense of physical and emotional well being referred to by drug users as the "high".

EXCIPIENT INGREDIENT:
A substance (usually without drug action) added to medications to give form, consistency, flavor, etc.

EXCRETION:
Process by which a drug and its metabolic products are eliminated from the body.

FETAL ALCOHOL SYNDROME:
Developmental defects occurring in offspring of alcoholic women.

FLASHBACK:
Spontaneous recurrence of an experience identical with a chemical effect in the absence of any chemical.

FLUORINATED:
Addition of a fluorine atom to a basic molecular structure.

FREON:
Liquid fluorocarbons used mainly as refrigerants, coolants, or aerosol propellants.

GOUT:
A metabolic disease (sometimes induced by alcoholism) characterized by recurrent attacks of arthritis, especially of the great toe.

HALF-LIFE (BIOLOGIC):
The amount of time it takes for the body to eliminate 50% of the drug molecules from the blood stream.

HALLUCINATION:
A subjective perception of something non-existent.

HYDROLYSIS:
Chemical reaction which results in breaking into smaller molecules and release of water.

HYDROXYLATION:
In metabolism of a chemical, addition of an -OH (hydroxyl) group to a chemical to render it more water soluble for urinary excretion.

IDIOSYNCRATIC:
Peculiar, unexpected.

INHALANT:
A volatile substance which is introduced into the body via the lung.

IONIZED:
Essentially means existing in a more water soluble form.

KORSAKOFF'S PSYCHOSIS:
A nervous system disorder resulting in memory failure, confabulation, and sometimes hallucinations and agitation.

LD50:
Abbreviation representing the quantity of a chemical that is fatal to 50% of the test population.

LIMBIC SYSTEM:
A portion of the brain involved in emotional tone.

LIPID SOLUBILITY/WATER SOLUBILITY:
Characteristics which describe the ability to or degree to which a chemical will dissolve in fatty, or non-fatty substance or tissue.

LOOK-ALIKE:
An inert or less potent chemical which has been intentionally prepared to look like a well known form of a more powerful, expensive, or less available chemical. The look-alikes in use in any community depend on availability and local use patterns, e.g., diazepam for methaqualone or secobarbital.

MEMBRANES:
A thin layer of tissue (often made up of fat and protein complexes) separating one structure from another.

METABOLISM:
The various chemical reactions involved in the changing of a drug in the body, usually (although not always) from an active to an inactive compound.

MICROSOMAL ETHANOL OXIDIZING SYSTEM:
(MEOS) one pathway of ethanol metabolism. It is induceable and may be partially responsible for tolerance to alcohol.

MICROSOMES:
Protein structures in the cytoplasm involved in metabolism.

NAD:
(Nicotinamide-adenine dinucleotide) an energy co-factor necessary for many of the chemical reactions in the body to occur.

NARCOTIC ANALGESIC:
Any natural, or synthetic drug with pharmacologic actions which are similar to morphine. (synonym: opioid).

NEURON:
A nerve cell.

NEUROTRANSMITTER:
Chemicals which transmit nerve messages across synaptic clefts.

NITRITES:
Class of compounds derived from nitrous acid which act as potent vasodilators.

NUCLEUS:
Spherical body in a cell which controls cell growth, metabolism, and reproduction.

NYSTAGMUS:
Oscillation of the eyeballs.

OVER DOSE:
Intake in excess of specified quantity of a therapeutic agent.

PARASYMPATHETIC NERVOUS SYSTEM:
The part of the autonomic nervous system which opposes the effects of the sympathetic nervous system. Generally, it tends to stimulate digestive secretions, slowing of the heart, and dilating blood vessels. It is often referred to as the "feed and breed" system.

PARASYMPATHOMIMETIC:
Denoting stimulation of parasympathetic nerve action.

PARASYMPATHOLYTIC:
An agent that annuls or antagonizes the effects of parasympathetic nerve action.

PERCEPTUAL DISTORTER:
A chemical which has the ability to cause altered states of perception, and altered states of thought and feeling. (synonomous with psychedelics, hallucinogens).

PERIPHERAL NERVOUS SYSTEM:
The part of the nervous system, outside of the central nervous system, including sensory and motor nerves.

PHARMACOLOGY:
The branch of basic science which deals with the actions on biological systems, usually human, of chemicals used in medicine for diagnostic and therapeutic purposes.

PHOSPHORYLATION:
The addition of a PO_4 (phosphate) chemical group to an organic compound.

PLACENTAL BARRIER:
The lipid membranes which impede transfer of many substances from the blood into the placenta.

PLASMA PROTEINS:
Protein portions of the circulating blood, or serum.

PSEUDOHALLUCINATION:
As opposed to hallucinations — unreal images which the victum can distinguish as being unreal.

PSYCHOACTIVE CHEMICALS:
Drugs which affect the mind.

PSYCHOMOTOR STIMULANT:
A chemical which excites the central nervous system.

RE-UPTAKE:
Process of active transport of neuro-transmitters from extracellular fluid (synapse) to cytoplasmic mobile pool (presynaptic terminal).

RECEPTOR SITE (DRUG):
A portion of a cell which participates in drug-cell interactions to initiate a drug action.

REM (RAPID EYE MOVEMENT):
The rapid, jerky movements of the eyes which occur during certain stages of the sleep cycle when dreams occur.

REM REBOUND:
The excessive REM sleep which occurs, along with nightmares, when a person has been denied REM sleep for a long period of time.

RETICULAR ACTIVATING SYSTEM (RAS):
Nerves located in the brain stem involved in wakefullness.

RHINOPHYMA:
A painless increase in size of the lower part of the nose.

SEDATIVE HYPNOTIC DRUG:
Chemicals which depress the central nervous system.

SOCIOPATHIC:
Describing the characteristic of being poorly adjusted to society due to quarrelsome, rebellious, aggressive, and/or immoral attitudes.

SOLVENT:
A substance (usually liquid) which is capable of dissolving another substance.

SPIDER ANGIOMAS:
A star-shaped swelling due to dilation of the blood vessels.

STATUS EPILEPTICUS:
A condition where major attacks of seizures follow after one another with little or no intermission.

STRAIGHT-CHAINED HYDROCARBON:
Chemicals composed of hydrogen and carbon which do not have branched or cyclic compounds.

SYMPATHETIC NERVOUS SYSTEM:
The portion of the autonomic nervous system which usually opposes the parasympathetic nervous system. It is sometimes referred to as the "fight or flight" system, and among other effects, dilates respiratory passages, increases blood flow to vital organs and decreases gastrointestinal activity.

SYMPATHETIC (ADRENERGIC):
Relating to nerve fibers that liberate adrenalin-like substances.

SYMPATHOLYTIC:
An agent that annuls or inhibits the effects of adrenergic stimulation.

SYMPATHOMIMETIC:
Denoting stimulation of adrenergic nerve action.

SYMPTOM RE-EMERGENCE:
After discontinuation of administration of a chemical, the re-occurance of disorders or symptoms which had been treated by that chemical.

SYNAPSE:
The place where a nerve impulse is transmitted from one neuron to another.

SYNERGISM:
The unpredictable enhancement of the effect of one chemical by the presence of another. The effect is more than could be expected from the combined amount of the two chemicals.

SYNESTHESIA:
The occurance of one type of stimulation evoking the sensation of another for example, hearing a sound resulting in the sensation of visualiz-
ing a color.

TACHYPHYLAXIS:
Rapid production of immunity to effects.

TETRAHYDROISOQUINOLINES:
Alkaloids chemically related to morphine which affect addictive behavior
in at least some laboratory animals.

TOLERANCE:
A biological or psychological phenomenon which results in a diminishing
or reduced effect on an individual from the same amount of some psychoactive chemical.

VOLATILE:
Capable of being easily vaporized at normal temperatures or pressures.

WERNICKE'S SYNDROME:
A mental disorder marked by memory loss, disorientation, and
confabulation.

WITHDRAWAL:
The signs and symptoms seen following decrease or cessation of a drug
on which the user has become physically dependent.

BIBLIOGRAPHY

BIBLIOGRAPHY

Abramowicz, M., et al. "Interactions of drugs with alcohol." *The Medical Letter.* 23(7):33-4, 1981.

Allen, A., and Clark, T. "Amphetamines." *Texas Medicine.* 69:95-8, 1973.

Becker, C.E., et al. *Alcohol As a Drug.* Baltimore, William and Wilkins Co., 1974.

Borruso, R. "Cocaine, a review." *US Pharmacist.* Sept. 1978: 78+

Boyd, J.R., et al. *Drug Facts and Comparisons, 1983 edition.* St. Louis, J.B. Lippincott Co., 1982.

Cohen, S. "Amphetamine abuse." *JAMA.* 231(4): 414-5, 1975.

Ellinwood, E.H., and Kilbey, M.M. *Cocaine and Other Stimulants.* New York, Plenum Press, 1977.

Geokas, M.C., et al. "Ethanol, the liver, and the gastrointestinal tract." *Annals of Internal Medicine.* 95(2):198-211, 1981.

Goldstein, A., et al. *Principles of Drug Action: The Basis of Pharmacology* 2nd edition. New York, John Wiley and Sons, 1974.

Goodman, L.S. and Gilman, A. *The Pharmacoligal Basis of Therapeutics* 5th edition. New York, Macmillan Publishing Co., 1975.

Graham, J.O.P., et al. *Cannabis and Health.* New York, Academic Press, 1976.

Johnson, C.D., et al. "Alcohol and sex." *Heart and Lung.* 12(1):93-7, 1983.

Knoben, J.E., and Anderson, P.O. *Handbook of Clinical Drug Data* 5th edition. Hamilton, Ill., Drug Intelligence Publications, Inc., 1983.

Lemberger, L., and Rubin, A. *Physiologic Disposition of Drugs of Abuse.* New York, Spectrum Publications, Inc., 1976

Littauer, U.Z., et al. *Neurotransmitters and Their Receptors,* New York, John Wiley and Sons, 1980.

Lowinson, J.H., and Ruiz, P. *Substance Abuse: Clinical Problems and Perspectives.* Baltimore, Williams and Wilkens, 1981.

Manning, F.C. "Methylphenidate" *Texas Medicine.* 69:89-90, June 1973.

Marks, V., and Wright, J., et al. "Metabolic effects of alcohol." *Clinics in Endocrinology and Metabolism.* 7(2), July 1978.

Nicholi, A.M. "The nontherapeutic use of psychoactive drugs, a modern epidemic." *NEJM.* 308(16):925-33, 1983.

Peterson, R.C. *Marijuana Research Findings; 1976.* Rockville, MD., U.S. Department of Health, Education, and Welfare, 1977.

Pradhan, S.M., and Dutta, S.N. *Drug Abuse: Clinical and Basic Aspects.* St. Louis, C.V. Mosby Co., 1977.

Sankar, D.V.S. *LSD- A Total Study.* Westbury, N.Y., PJD Publications, 1975.

Smith, H.M. "Marijuana and public health." *MD* Feb. 1983:137-52.

Wilford, B.B. *Drug Abuse, A Guide For the Primary Care Physician.* Chicago, AMA, 1981.

Zuska, Joseph J. "Wounds without a cause." *American College of Surgeons Bulletin*, October, 1981.